Testimonials fo
and Detoxing for Life

Due to a huge amount of stress over the years as a priest and fire and police chaplain, I had gained about fifty pounds, almost without realizing it. Facing hip replacement and feeling tired like an old man, I tried all kinds of diets hoping that would help. I'd lose some weight, but I kept gaining it back. Then I discovered Cherie's juicing and cleansing program. I have now lost about forty-one pounds! Sometimes I replace two meals with juice and that's all I want. It's taken away my cravings — no more desire for junk foods, high-carb foods, or desserts. No more struggling! My energy level has shot up and people are always commenting on the weight I've lost and how great my skin looks. I no longer feel twenty years older than my age, but twenty years younger!

— Father Tryphon, age 61

When I was feeling hopeless about my hypothyroid condition and the extra twenty pounds I was carrying, my naturopathic doctor told me I had to do a detox. He said it was the only way to get my body back in balance and off of thyroid medication. So, I did a serious detox with mostly raw food and the juice diet, along with some supplements, and finally, after trying for years, I dropped twelve pounds effortlessly in just months. It made a believer out of me! I didn't realize that toxins are stored in fat and that the body holds onto fat for our protection. Get rid of the toxins; get rid of the fat. I don't think I could have lost the weight without going to mostly raw foods and juice and cleansing. I didn't know that detoxing was such a critical part of shedding stubborn fat.

— Trudy, 49

At age thirty-nine, I was so unhealthy I thought I'd be dead before I turned fifty. I felt sick all the time, tired, and had severe pain in my abdomen and lower back. At forty-one, I was diagnosed with colon cancer, which spread to my liver, lungs, and other areas of my body. The doctors didn't give me hope of recovery. That was when I found Cherie's juicing and cleansing program. First I went on the three-week alkalizing diet. Four days into the colon cleanse, my body got rid of a mass about the size of my fist. I continued to go to the clinic for monitoring, and, surprisingly, my tumor markers repeatedly went down and down. At the same time, I started feeling better and better. My energy returned. My pain went away. And I started looking healthier. I'm now forty-seven, and my doctors finally pronounced me *cancer free!* I've never felt better in my life! Recently, I ran up a flight of stairs like a teenager. When I look in the mirror, I'm truly amazed at how much younger I look. Just the other day a lady told me I looked about thirty-seven. I know my great health, youthful appearance, and my life is due to a program of juicing, alkalizing and cleansing.   —*Barbara, 47*

I've lost about twenty-five pounds since I started my juicing, raw foods diet, and cleanse program. A year before, I'd set a goal to lose twelve pounds and just couldn't do it. Then I went on the juicing and raw foods program to focus on optimum health because I was diagnosed with breast cancer. Surprisingly, the weight just fell off. I eat a lot of food—all good food, and a high percentage of it is raw. And I'm not hungry at all. I have lots of energy. But the best news is that my tumor markers have fallen to half the score I started with. And I feel better than I have in years. I look younger, my hair is thicker, and my skin is clear.   —*Nancy, 60*

Juicing, Fasting, and Detoxing for Life

Juicing, Fasting, and Detoxing for Life

Unleash the Healing Power of
Fresh Juices and Cleansing Diets

◆

CHERIE CALBOM, MS
WITH JOHN CALBOM, MA

**WELLNESS
CENTRAL**

NEW YORK   BOSTON

The information and advice herein is not intended to replace the services of trained health professionals, or be a substitute for medical advice. You are advised to consult with your health care professional with regard to matters relating to your health, and in particular regarding matters that may require diagnosis or medical attention.

Wellness Central
Hachette Book Group USA
237 Park Avenue
New York, NY 10017

Visit our Web site at www.HachetteBookGroupUSA.com.

Wellness Central is an imprint of Grand Central Publishing.
The Wellness Central name and logo are trademarks of Hachette Book Group USA, Inc.

Printed in the United States of America

First Edition: July 2008
10 9 8 7 6 5 4 3 2 1

Library of Congress Cataloging-in-Publication Data

Calbom, Cherie.
    Juicing, fasting, and detoxing for life : unleash the healing power of fresh juices and cleansing diets / Cherie Calbom with John Calbom. — 1st ed.
        p. cm.
    Includes index.
    ISBN-13: 978-0-446-58137-0
    ISBN-10: 0-446-58137-2
    1. Detoxification (Health).   2. Fruit juices.   3. Vegetable juices.
4. Fasting.   I. Calbom, John.   II. Title.
    RA784.5.C35 2008
    613—dc22   2007043715

Book design by Stratford Publishing Services, a TexTech business

Contents

Introduction

Would you like to be healthy, happy, and energetic? Want to look younger and more vibrant? How about losing some weight? Or do you need help healing your body? If you said yes to any of these questions, rest assured. The programs in *Juicing, Fasting, and Detoxing for Life* have helped thousands of people lose weight, get rid of cellulite, look healthier, soften wrinkles and lines, gain energy, restore health, prevent disease, and feel years younger.

If you have a health issue, this can be your opportunity to discover not only what contributed to your ill health, but what will enable you to become healthier than before and live an exciting, fulfilling life of purpose. Even if you don't have any particular ailments, you can experience more energy and greater vitality along with disease prevention by using the programs such as juicing, short juice fasts, and periodic detoxes for various organs of the body.

I first wrote about juicing in 1992 in my best-selling book *Juicing for Life*. Nearly two million people have read *Juicing for Life*, and my sequel, *The Juice Lady's Guide to Juicing for Health*. Exciting testimonies have poured in from people all across America and around the world whose lives have changed for the better when they started juicing, cleansed their body, and changed their diet. The "live foods" I recommend such as fresh vegetable juices, veggie smoothies, and raw foods give life to the body. And the yummy recipes allow for delicious and varied menus. I'm convinced the juicing and cleansing programs I've developed have saved my life by helping me recover from debilitating illness and injury. And I know they'll make a big difference for you, too.

The programs in *Juicing, Fasting, and Detoxing for Life* go far beyond salads and V8 juice. In fact, juices that are canned or bottled have been pasteurized, which means that many of their life-giving nutrients such as enzymes and vitamins have been killed in the process. And while these processed options are better than soda pop, they fall quite short when compared with freshly made juice. But there's another important reason to drink fresh juice. It's broken down into an easily absorbable form, which makes it superior to even eating whole vegetables, when it comes to absorbing vitamins, minerals, and enzymes. Plus, you'd probably never eat in one day all the vegetables you'd juice. Live foods like fresh juice, veggie smoothies, green salads and other raw foods, along with a diet of whole foods offer an abundance of nutrients. They make your body feel alive!

The programs in *Juicing, Fasting, and Detoxing for Life* include short juice fasts and specific cleanse programs that act similar to spa treatments on the inside. They're somewhat like a housecleaning crew for your organs and fluids, on down to your cells. Juicing, fasting, and detoxing can help you get well if you're ill and make you even healthier if you're well — perhaps more vibrant and energetic than you ever thought possible. And that means when you lose weight using these programs, you'll look healthier — and you won't drown or look washed out as many people do on other plans.

There are many detox programs on the market, and many focus on items to purchase. Very few programs have detailed menu plans with plenty of delicious recipes that make it easy to follow and don't require a huge expense. Though a few of my cleanse programs need certain herbs or other cleanse agents to make them the most effective, many of the programs can simply be followed with recipes you prepare.

In the chapters that follow, you'll find the plans that turned my life around — from illness, debilitation, and disability to good health and a desire to help others be well. I want to share with you my own journey to health and wholeness to encourage you. If I could get well and stay healthy, there's hope and the opportunity for you to do the same.

A Health Crisis

Though I'd never been particularly healthy as a child and adolescent, I encountered a true health crisis when I turned thirty. I developed a severe case of chronic fatigue syndrome that forced me to quit my job in Hollywood and move home to Colorado with my father and stepmother. I was simply too sick and tired to do much more than lie around most of the time. I would often sleep twelve hours at a time and still feel tired when I got up. Severe fatigue became a way of life. There were mornings when I'd get up feeling so weak that I could barely walk down the hall. I felt as if I had a never-ending case of the flu with continual swollen glands and a low-grade fever. My body ached as if I'd just been bounced around in a washing machine. And I had a severe case of candidiasis along with parasite (determined by a stool test) and heavy metal toxicity (determined by a hair analysis). My life seemed hopeless.

I'd not been able to find a doctor who could give me anything to improve my health or any hope of feeling better. I finally went to a health food store and browsed around. I talked with employees and bought some health books. I discovered there *was* something I could do.

I totally changed my diet and started juicing every day. I eliminated all animal products, including dairy, along with all junk food, sugar, and wheat products. I started with a five-day juice fast. In the weeks that followed, I completed several other short juice fasts of two or three days and several cleansing programs. But instead of feeling better, I started feeling a little worse. Though I didn't understand the process at the time, I was *detoxing.* Detoxification is the process of removing from the body toxins, which are substances that are harmful or poisonous. They create irritating or injurious effects internally, undermining our health and stressing our biochemical and organ functions. Removing them doesn't happen on a wide scale without our assistance through nutritional intervention, cleansing programs, and dietary changes.

Family members were skeptical about my self-designed health journey, but I forged on with my whole foods diet, juicing, and cleansing programs. I also saw a reflexologist (a person who massages feet and applies pressure to certain parts of the foot for healing). He suggested I try a gallbladder flush because of pain when pressure was applied to a specific area of my foot. The gallbladder detox produced rather astounding results and I did get a little better. But I still often felt sick and tired.

Then one day, totally unexpected, I woke up feeling brand-new — with energy to spare. I wanted to go jogging. That was a first. I'd made a significant turn for the better, and though my new health seemed to suddenly appear, it had been building for quite a while. I'd been on my health program for about three months. And I thought, "Wow! That was the greatest cure on earth." I realized that freshly made vegetable juices, veggie smoothies, lots of raw foods, periodic cleansing, and a nutritious, whole foods diet was a lifestyle I could follow for life to produce the health I wanted. I also realized there were foods I needed to let go of, like sweets, flour products such as bread and pasta, and dairy products, so I could maintain my high level of wellness.

Armed with a juicer, a new lifestyle, and an exciting set of goals, I returned to Southern California and my friends. For nearly a year, it was *ten steps forward* with renewed, sparkling health and more energy and stamina than I'd ever remembered.

Then, all of a sudden, I took a *giant* step back.

Another Crisis

I was house-sitting in a lovely Southern California neighborhood for vacationing family friends and working on my first book. A burglar broke into their home one night. I was shocked to wake up around three a.m.

and see a strange young man in the bedroom. Instead of running, he attacked, beating me repeatedly with a pipe, yelling, "Now you are dead!" and then choking me unconscious. I felt my spirit leave, floating up and out of my body. Then all was still. I sensed I was traveling, at what seemed like the speed of light, through black space, with twinkling lights in the distance. Suddenly, however, I was back in my body, outside the house, screaming for help. I don't know how I got there.

I suffered serious injuries to my head, neck, back, and right hand, with multiple head wounds and part of my scalp torn from my head. I also incurred numerous cracked teeth that resulted in several root canals and crowns. But my right hand sustained the most severe injuries, with two knuckles crushed to mere bone fragments that had to be held together by metal pins, and six months after the attack, I still couldn't use it. The cast I wore, with bands holding up my ring finger that was almost torn from my hand (it had remained attached by only a small portion of skin), looked like something from a science-fiction movie. I felt and looked worse than hopeless, with the top of my head shaved, red, swollen eyes, a gash on my face, a useless right hand, terrorizing fear, and barely enough energy to get dressed when I woke up.

I decided I'd be a survivor, not a victim. So I went to work on getting well again. This time, it took every

ounce of my will, deep spiritual work, alternative medical help, extra vitamins and minerals, juicing, emotional
release, forgiveness of the attacker, and numerous detox
programs to heal physically, mentally, and emotionally.

I met a nutritionally minded physician who had
healed his own slow-mending broken bones with lots of
vitamins and minerals; he gave me vitamin cocktail IVs.
Juicing, cleansing, nutritional supplements, a nearly perfect diet, and prayer, along with physical therapy helped
my bones and other injuries heal.

After following this regimen for several months,
what my hand surgeon said would be impossible became
real — a fully restored, fully functional hand. He'd told
me I'd never use my right hand again, and that it wasn't
even possible to put in plastic knuckles because of its
poor condition. But my knuckles did indeed re-form
and function of my hand returned. A day came when
he told me I was completely healed, and though the doctor admitted he didn't believe in miracles, he did say,
"You're the closest thing I've seen to one."

Equally important in the restorative process was the
healing of my soul — a place no one could determine the
degree of injury. I experienced healing from the painful memories and trauma of the attack through prayer,
laying-on of hands, and deep emotional healing work. It
seemed like endless buckets of tears had been pent-up
in my soul from old wounds, such as my mother's death

when I was six, my grandfather's death when I was nine, a tragedy concerning my dad when I was thirteen, along with the attack. All that pain needed release. Forgiveness and letting go came in stages and was an integral part of my total healing. I had to be honest about what I really felt and willing to face the pain and toxic emotions stored inside and let them go. But, finally, I was free. A time came when I could celebrate the Fourth of July (the anniversary of the attack) without fear.

Finally, I knew more peace and health than I ever thought possible. I experienced what it was to feel *whole* — complete, not damaged, broken, wounded, or impaired, but truly healed and restored to wholeness in body, soul, and spirit. And I knew there was a purpose for my life — a reason I had lived. I could help others find their way to wholeness.

You Can Enjoy Vibrant Health

Because of my health struggles and the long journey to wholeness by a road of trial and error, I wrote this book for you — wherever you're at in your pursuit of good health and vitality. You may be healthy and just want to gain a little more energy, lose a few pounds, and bolster your immune system so you don't get colds or flu as much. You may have a health condition you want to improve. Or you may have a life-threatening illness or serious injury and you want to do your part in getting well. Whatever it is you want to achieve, I know that you can make significant improvements in your health by following the programs in *Juicing, Fasting, and Detoxing for Life.*

I'm sharing with you what I've learned on my path to health and wholeness, as well as what I've studied in scientific research and in earning a graduate degree in nutrition, along with what I've discovered through years of counseling people regarding nutrition and their health. I've seen hundreds of people achieve near perfect health and get rid of a host of ailments, aches and pains, and even life-threatening diseases through juicing and following the various cleanse programs in this book. There's no magic bullet in this process — it's all about giving your body what it needs to heal and stay healthy along with getting rid of what hinders the healing process. As you remove toxicity, which interferes with health and healing, and give your body an abundance of life-giving nutrients like those found in fresh juice, your body can do what it was designed to — heal and stay healthy and trim.

In the chapter on mental and emotional cleansing, my husband, John, shares the knowledge he's gained about mental and emotional detox. Through his graduate work in counseling psychology and over thirty years of working with groups and individuals regarding the care and healing of the soul, he's gained tremendous insights on letting go of mental and emotional toxicity and how to restore the soul.

Keep in mind that as you embark on your journey to vibrant health it will take trust, patience, and endurance along with action to get good results. Restoration and preservation of your health comes with time and persistence. If you stick with the programs in *Juicing, Fasting, and Detoxing for Life*, you will have a healthier body and soul. Your body was intended to function well. If you have physical ailments, remember that your body was designed to heal. It's important to provide the best internal environment possible so it can do its work of healing. Remember, it's taken a while to get to where you're at, so it may take a while to correct your health issues. Take heart! You'll reach your goal if you don't give up. And while you're on your journey to vibrant health, be aware that any problems you face can be part of the weave of your new life of wholeness, vitality, and purpose—the purpose for which you were created.

You can begin your journey today by taking the first step—whatever that may be for you. Maybe you need to purchase a juicer or just simply go shopping for fresh, organic produce, or make a decision that you're going to do things that are really good for your body from this day forward. Whatever you need to do to get started, take that step today.

Juicing and Cleansing Programs That Get Results

Make fresh vegetable juicing a part of your routine — it can be life changing! Fast occasionally. Some people like to vegetable-juice fast one day a week; others choose to fast one or two days each month or once a quarter. Once or twice a year, or optimally, once a quarter, cleanse your colon, liver and gallbladder, and kidneys. If it makes sense to change the oil and filters in your car regularly, doesn't it make sense to cleanse your body's filter systems? Be sure to stick with the cleanse programs even if you feel a little worse initially. As you clear toxins from your body, you may not feel so great before you feel better. But when you've completed the detox programs, you'll feel like a new person.

The same goes for cleansing the soul. As you clear mental and emotional toxicity from your mind and emotions, you may have to face unpleasant memories and old wounds, emotional pain may surface, and buried memories may be revealed. But the results are worth the effort. Nothing can compare with deep peace, joy, and a healthier body that comes from a balanced soul.

You'll find the chapters in *Juicing, Fasting, and Detoxing for Life* to be informative and easy to follow. In chapter one you'll discover the secrets of vibrant health. Chapter two introduces you to the world of juicing and gives you guidelines for using fresh juice for vitality, energy, healing, and detoxing your body. It also gives you lots of tips for purchasing a juicer that's easy to use and clean; a blender won't work for juicing, but you'll use one for smoothies and cold soups. Chapter three tells you all about the benefits of fasting and how to begin with a one- to three-day vegetable juice fast that will greatly accelerate any weight loss or health program you choose. Chapter four gives you an overview of detoxification and explains why it's so important to your health. Various detoxification protocols follow in chapters five through seven with juices, veggie smoothies, cold soups, raw foods, and supplements for the Colon Cleanse, Liver and Gallbladder Cleanse, Kidney Cleanse, along with various specialized cleanses for *Candida albicans*, parasites, and heavy metals. Chapter eight guides you through detoxing your mind and emotions. Chapter nine follows with an A to Z guide that gives you a list of the foods that are highest in nutrients from vitamin A to zinc. And the last chapter gives you dozens of delicious juice and veggie smoothie recipes.

John and I have learned through personal experience that proper cleansing of the organs of elimination can happen only through specific plans designed to promote "housecleaning" in each organ. We've completed numerous cleansing programs and have seen encouraging results each time. If you're ill, or highly motivated and have the time, you can go directly from one cleanse to the next. Or, you can pace yourself with one cleanse at a time with space in between.

And if you work away from home, you can still do the cleanse programs. Countless people have completed specific cleanses and short juice fasts and were still able to work outside their home and even enjoy a social life. It takes some planning ahead and preparation before each day so you can take what you need to work. You can also plan for certain social events by eating ahead of time and ordering sparkling water with lemon or lime or herbal tea at the event. You can choose what will work for you at restaurants by asking the chef to prepare special all-vegetable salads or vegetable or vegan dishes. The goal is to fit the detox programs into your busy lifestyle and make them work. If you have a demanding or stressful job, and you can try only one cleanse program when you have a few days off or a one-day vegetable-juice fast on a weekend day, this is a good start. Whatever positive changes you make, it will move you toward better health and give your overworked systems of elimination a much-needed rest so they can cleanse and rejuvenate.

A Healthier, More Vibrant Life Awaits You

When you complete these juicing, fasting, and cleansing programs, you'll have changed your internal environment. You should feel lighter, healthier, and happier. And as a friend of mine said recently, "You'll feel like smiling all the time!" You'll have more energy to enjoy each and every day. And you'll have the best chance of preventing common and even serious illnesses. If you're ill, you'll give your body the greatest chance to heal. Best of all, you'll have discovered a way of life that will help you feel and look alive and vibrant each and every day. A healthier, more balanced life truly does await you!

CHAPTER ONE

The Secrets of Vibrant Health

Healthy, trim, energetic, and full of life! That's what you can be when you incorporate the secrets of juicing, fasting, and cleansing, along with whole, organic foods into your lifestyle. You can easily make these wonderful steps to healing and vitality a part of your daily life. You're about to discover a program that really works. It's worked for us and for thousands of other people. It can work for you.

If you're feeling sick and tired much of the time despite your best efforts at living a healthy life, don't be discouraged. I'll help you turn that around. Maybe you've been struggling to lose weight and just can't seem to get it off or keep it off — you lose a few pounds only to gain them back, plus a few more. Or maybe you're feeling sluggish and tired; fatigue is a constant reminder that something's amiss. Perhaps you have frequent headaches, back pain, or pain elsewhere in your body. Your sleep may be disturbed or you may wake up in the morning still feeling tired. Your digestion may be off kilter — you experience gas, bloating, or constipation. Your immune system may not be up to par and, consequently, you experience frequent colds, flu, infections, or sinus problems. All these symptoms could be signals that your body is in need of the supernutrition found in fresh juice and the detox programs within these pages.

Whatever your health challenges or goals may be, you can benefit from the life-giving nutrients in freshly made juice and raw foods. You can get an energy and vitality boost from short juice fasts. And, because your system may be overloaded and overworked trying to clear out excess toxicity that has accumulated in your cells, tissues, and organs, you could greatly benefit from the detox programs in *Juicing, Fasting, and Detoxing for Life.*

Detoxing for Radiant Health

Research shows that the average person is exposed to thousands of toxins and environmental pollutants on a daily basis, more than ever before in history, and all this toxic waste takes a toll on the body. The U.S. Environmental Protection Agency (EPA) reported that eighty-seven thousand new chemicals are being produced every year. Without a periodic program of detoxing, it's almost impossible to stay on top of eliminating all this stuff and keep your body in a state of health. But take heart. I'll show you how to use juicing, fasting, and detoxing programs to systematically clean out your cells, tissues, and organs of elimination and jump-start your health right away.

Detox programs and products are showing up nearly everywhere these days, as people discover how they improve health. There are books and magazines that continue to promote the newest detox plans. Numerous health spas offer special detox wraps, natural mineral springs (which promote detox), and cleansing programs to revamp your health and vitality. Health food stores have huge displays of cleansing and detox products. And it seems that nearly everyone we talk to about detoxing has an opinion or a question about how to do it or how it will be of benefit.

Unfortunately, many products and plans either don't work or are difficult to use. Some of the programs require little or no effort on your part; they say just take the product or try this quick-fix treatment and you're done — your nagging symptoms will all disappear. Keep in mind that there are no quick fixes. It took a number of years to get to this point, and it will take a while to get it cleared up. But while it requires time, patience, and some discipline, it's not difficult. And the rewards are huge.

Many people tell me they eat a reasonably healthy diet, get some exercise on a regular basis, and don't eat bad stuff like junk food or desserts — at least not too often. Some people ask, "But isn't it good enough just to eat lots of fruits and vegetables, drink some vegetable juice like V8, buy organic produce most of the time, and try not to eat too much junk?" That's a fair maintenance program. But to get rid of toxins and keep your body healthy, you need to detox it periodically. And that doesn't happen when you're eating regular meals your body has to concentrate on digesting all day long. Consequently, it doesn't have much time for cleanup and repair, let alone time to move out toxins that are tucked away in fat cells and other spaces. To accomplish detoxification, you need to juice fast once in a while and utilize the colon, liver and gallbladder, and kidney cleanses periodically. This is the best way to stay trim, fit, and healthy or to get well again. And it's possible to accomplish this in the real world without being overly obsessed. It can even be fun once you get the hang of it.

Periodic detoxing can help you get rid of irritating toxins that do harm in the body and stubborn fat like belly fat. The key word here is "periodic." I'm not telling you to live on only juices, raw foods, and herbs for the rest of your life, but to periodically detoxify your body with the programs in this book, to juice most days of the week, and to eat a high percentage of your food raw.

Once you've completed a detox program, you can follow up with a maintenance program of whole foods, plenty of fresh vegetable juices, raw foods, purified water, regular exercise, and emotional and spiritual cleansing. I'll show you how to make it work no matter how busy or complicated your life might be. And if you're short on funds, I've got many programs you can put together inexpensively.

Since it's nearly impossible to meet your health and wellness goals without doing something to counteract the influences of ever-increasing toxicity, whether it's physical, emotional, mental, or spiritual, you must tackle the negativity with determination. Nevertheless, you don't want to be compulsively regimented about food and dieting, or anything else for that matter. I'm not advocating overdoing it to the point of making your eating habits a source of stress or fear, which will only make you feel worse, because you're probably already trying to fit a lot into your busy life. Some people tend to go overboard on health and dieting. They become food police for themselves and others, frequently driving themselves into a state of stress and exhaustion in their pursuit of perfect health. This can undo all the hard work of getting healthy. And so, the point of this book is to guide you toward a balanced lifestyle, by making juicing a way of life, helping you find short-term cleansing programs that work for you, and providing useful tips, delicious recipes, and support to keep you on track along the way.

Why You Need to Detox

Even if you moved to a deserted island in the middle of the South Pacific and ate only organic coconuts and vegetables grown in your own garden, you still could not be sure you were totally safe from pollution. The air you breathe might have picked up radiation from half-way around the globe; the fish you caught could be contaminated with mercury from a far-off shore; the water might not be safe to drink due to acid rain.

The reality is that we live on a planet that is polluted. The air we breathe is loaded with invisible pollutants, our food supplies are often toxic due to pesticides and preservatives, and we can't trust the water supply due to water-treatment chemicals. We are exposed to thousands of toxins and chemicals in our homes, yards, work places, schools, on our highways, where we shop, in our sleep, and in the food we eat. It doesn't matter how old we are, what we do for a living, or even where we live. Environmental pollution is everywhere. These toxins include industrial chemicals, insecticides, pesticides, heavy metals, emissions from the burning of organic fuels, electromagnetic pollution, radiation, hormones and antibiotics used in animal farming, and food dyes, preservatives, and additives added to our food. We're bombarded with reactive molecules called free radicals that can damage our cells. The use of pharmaceutical and over-the-counter drugs results in side effects that can interact with other drugs and substances to cause further toxicity. Average people like you and me are being inundated with thousands of chemicals whose names most of us can't pronounce and that are invisible to us, yet inevitably they take a toll on our bodies. The assault on our bodies continues year after year, gradually weakening our organs and compromising our immune systems — our bodies' natural defense.

Toxic chemicals affect every aspect of our bodies in some way — cells, tissues, and organs become overloaded with waste. Fortunately, we are equipped with organs of elimination and detoxification to clear away the accumulation of these pollutants. But when our organs become overwhelmed with too much work, a buildup of toxicity occurs and we become more and more fatigued, mentally fogged, and susceptible to sickness. *Juicing, Fasting, and Detoxing for Life* shows you what you can do to assist your body in managing this onslaught from the environment and how to choose good health habits that will strengthen and protect you. A strong, healthy body can resist toxic overload and disease, so there's great incentive to become stronger, healthier, and more resistant.

Some Startling Effects of Toxicity

Many studies and reports link environmental pollution to the state of our health. Chemicals that were designed to enhance our lives were introduced into our environment over fifty years ago, but in the past half century hundreds of them have been shown to be either highly toxic and carcinogenic, or at least troublesome and irritating to our complex biological systems. It leaves us wondering what happened between what was supposed to make our lives better but instead is making us sick.

Less than 10 percent of all the chemicals in our environment have been even partially evaluated for safety. It's difficult to know exactly how many of them are actually harmful or highly carcinogenic and could damage our health, the health of our children, and the health of our planet. Environmental toxins disrupt normal metabolic functioning of the body, which over time can lead to poor quality of life, and have been linked to conditions such as chronic fatigue syndrome, fibromyalgia, autoimmune disorders, inflammatory diseases, infertility, and cancer.

Better Choices for Better Health

Now that we recognize that we live in a polluted world, what can we do to protect ourselves against this onslaught? Obviously, the first line of defense is to avoid toxins as much as possible. Although we can't avoid all exposure to environmental chemicals, especially those that we breathe in the air, we do have many and varied choices about what we put in our mouths and on our bodies, spray in our houses and on our lawns, use for cleaning products, and apply as cosmetics.

When it comes to water, we can use purified for drinking and food preparation to avoid the hidden sources of pollution. Make sure to use purified water for soup, coffee, tea, and ice cubes as well. And healthy food choices are something we can make each and every day. We can choose whole, unprocessed, organic foods grown without pesticides and chemical fertilizers. When choosing animal products, we can look for cage-free eggs and cage-free poultry and grass-fed beef, raised without hormones and antibiotics.

"What am I supposed to do?" a friend asked in frustration. "If the world is so toxic and there is no escape, why even try? Maybe I should just eat all the hamburgers, French fries, and chocolate chip cookies I want!" Well, that's certainly not the answer. We can make good choices and avoid some of the more flagrant sources of poisons, such as junk food, fried food, refined carbs, high-fat and high-sugar foods, and packaged items with preservatives. We can avoid pesticides and insecticides that are made for home and garden. We can say no to vaccinations, some of which still contain thimerosal, a mercury-containing organic compound that is widely used as a preservative in a number of biological and drug products, including vaccines. (This preservative could be especially harmful for babies and children and, though unproven, has been linked to autism. Before you get any vaccinations for yourself or your children, make sure they have no thimerosal or any other harmful preservatives. Why be a test case for a mercury-based product?) We can avoid mercury toxicity by asking our dentists to remove all amalgam fillings (silver-colored fillings containing mercury) and replace them with safer alternatives.

The use of pharmaceutical drugs often causes side effects that are worse than the conditions they are designed to treat, which then requires additional drugs to counteract the negative side effects of the first one, further taxing our bodies. We can get second opinions from doctors who specialize in natural medicine and search for nontoxic natural remedies whenever possible. We can also be very thoughtful about the use of over-the-counter drugs and search out natural remedies first. Although over-the-counter drugs are widely used, they present another source of toxicity.

How Toxic Are You?

Here is a quiz you can take to find out how toxic your environment is and how toxic you may be.

QUESTIONS	ANSWERS	POINTS
1. Do you currently smoke?	yes/no	5
2. Have you been a smoker for more than three years?	yes/no	3
3. Do you have silver mercury fillings?	yes/no	4
4. Do you regularly use household chemicals for cleaning, disinfecting, deodorizing, carpet cleaning, oven cleaning, stain removals?	yes/no	2
5. Have you had a root canal?	yes/no	3
6. Do you drink unfiltered water?	yes/no	2
7. Do you live in an urban environment?	yes/no	3
8. Do you consume alcohol?	yes/no	3
9. Do you use antiperspirants, nonorganic cosmetics, skin care products, or hair dye?	yes/no	2 (ea)

HAVE YOU EVER LIVED:

10. within ten miles of a nuclear power plant?	yes/no	4

(Continued)

QUESTIONS	ANSWERS	POINTS
11. within five miles of a toxic waste dump?	yes/no	5
12. near a farm where aerial pesticides are used?	yes/no	5
13. on a farm where pesticides are sprayed?	yes/no	5
14. Do you have asbestos in your house, workplace, or school?	yes/no	3
15. Do you consume fast foods?	yes/no	2
16. Have you ever worked professionally with pesticides or chemicals?	yes/no	5
17. Do you use pesticide on your residential lawn or garden?	yes/no	3
18. Do you have your clothes cleaned with professional dry-cleaning?	yes/no	1
19. Has your home been treated for termites in the past ten years?	yes/no	1
20. Do you consume nonorganically grown fruits and vegetables?	yes/no	2
21. Do you live in an area where the ground is known to contain radon gas?	yes/no	3
22. Do you eat in restaurants more than twice a week?	yes/no	2

23. Do you have wall-to-wall carpeting (unless nontoxic)? yes/no 2

24. Do you cook food in a microwave oven? yes/no 2

25. Do you spend less than fifteen minutes outdoors each day? yes/no 2

26. Do you have an energy-efficient house that rarely gets fresh air within? yes/no 2

27. Do you travel by air at least once a month? yes/no 2

DO YOU EXHIBIT ANY OF THE FOLLOWING SYMPTOMS?:

28. feel fatigued for no apparent reason yes/no 2

29. feel lifeless, depressed yes/no 2

30. feel light-headedness from time to time yes/no 1

31. have difficulty thinking clearly yes/no 1

32. suffer from aches and pains for no apparent reason yes/no 3

33. occasionally feel irritable for no reason yes/no 2

34. sometimes feel anxious for no reason yes/no 2

35. sometimes experience shortness of breath for no apparent reason yes/no 2

(*Continued*)

QUESTIONS	ANSWERS	POINTS

HAVE YOU TAKEN ANY OF THE FOLLOWING DRUGS?:
(1 POINT FOR LOW USAGE; 3 POINTS FOR HIGH USAGE)

36. prescription drugs	yes/no	1–3
37. painkillers/tranquilizers	yes/no	1–3
38. psychiatric drugs	yes/no	1–3
39. Ritalin	yes/no	1–3
40. over-the-counter drugs (aspirin, etc.)	yes/no	1–3
41. LSD	yes/no	1–3
42. heroin	yes/no	1–3
43. cocaine	yes/no	1–3
44. pot	yes/no	1–3
45. PCP	yes/no	1–3
46. methadone	yes/no	1–3
47. steroids	yes/no	1–3

Score:

Sum up the points for the questions where you answered yes:

1 to 15 points	You may have a low level of toxicity in your body.
15 to 25 points	You may have levels of toxicity in your body that could reduce your ability to stay healthy and think clearly.
26 to 40 points	You may have a level of toxicity in your body that causes you often to feel

fatigued, lethargic, mentally foggy, be susceptible to colds and flu.

41 to 50 points   You may have a high level of toxicity in your body that causes you to often get sick, feel mentally foggy, lethargic, fatigued, experience aches and pains, and be susceptible to disease.

>50 points   You could be experiencing extreme body toxicity, which could include all the symptoms listed above, make you susceptible to serious disease, and reduce the length and quality of your life.

If you scored even a few points on this quiz, this is an indication that you could benefit from cleansing your body.

Symptoms of Toxic Overload

- Headaches
- Constipation
- Bloating or gas
- Heartburn or indigestion
- Nausea
- Lethargy, tiredness, or fatigue
- Frequent colds and flu
- Puffiness or dark circles under eyes
- Arthritis, painful joints
- Congestion
- Shortness of breath
- Runny nose or constant sneezing
- Clogged sinuses
- Asthma or bronchitis
- Water retention
- Dark-colored, cloudy, strong-smelling urine
- Hives, rashes, or dry skin
- Pimples or rashes
- Cellulite
- Mood swings
- Anxiety, fear, or nervousness
- Sleeplessness
- Depression
- Confusion or poor concentration

What Happens When Toxicity Builds Up?

Most of us keep our floors swept and our clothes washed, and give our cars periodic oil changes. We understand the importance of cleaning and caring for our possessions, but we often neglect our own bodies. Our bodies are able to handle a certain amount of toxicity because we have immune systems and organs of elimination designed to clean out many of these toxic substances, but they can handle only so much before they become overwhelmed by the huge numbers of toxins that we ingest from the environment — air, water, and food.

The result is that substances that are not broken down and excreted are generally stored in the intestines, gallbladder, kidneys, liver, lymph, fat cells, and skin. The colon, which is designed to eliminate solid waste, can become sluggish and build up putrefaction. The liver can get congested and unable to properly filter the blood. The kidneys can get overwhelmed in their attempt to excrete toxic-laden urea. As a result, our systems are unable to function properly; nutrients are not absorbed well and poisons are reabsorbed into our bloodstream. Toxins are then stored in fat cells, they collect in other tissues and spaces between the cells, and they clog our lymphatic system. If the lymph isn't moving the debris out of our bodies, we can begin to feel sick. All this toxic buildup eventually affects our energy, mood, sleep, mental clarity, and immune function. We may feel sick, tired, and depressed. If we continue in this decline, we may get a disease.

What Detoxing Will Do for You

Detoxifying is another word for cleansing, which means to eliminate toxins. I'll use the words interchangeably. When you embark on a detox program, it may take some work at first, but the benefits are so astounding that it makes the effort worthwhile. You'll not only feel stronger and more energetic as a result, you'll start looking younger and more vibrant. You may look in the mirror one day and see fewer wrinkles, softer skin, or notice that dark circles or puffiness under your eyes are gone. Your skin will develop an underlying glow. Your hair will shine more and grow healthier and your nails will grow stronger.

People who have followed my detox programs also report greater mental clarity. "I can think straight again!" one client exclaimed. In most people there is a restored sense of well-being that may have eluded them for years. One friend said she reported to her doctor that she could never remember having a sense of well-being. His answer was to prescribe an antidepressant drug, which she refused. When I taught her about juicing, detoxing, and a whole foods diet, she reported back in a few weeks that she had finally gained that elusive sense of well-being she'd only read about.

When we give our bodies a rest from processing all the excesses, they're able to rebuild, repair, and strengthen organs and systems, which will protect us from disease. We won't be subject to every cold and flu that circulates, and our bodies can begin to heal from ailments that may have plagued us for years. Over the years I've received countless testimonies from people who have healed their bodies by juicing, fasting, and detoxing. One lady cleared up liver problems in one week with the liver cleanse. I've heard from people who have improved or healed a wide variety of ailments from fibromyalgia to cancer with the programs in *Juicing, Fasting, and Detoxing for Life.*

Detoxing also helps us lose weight. Vast amounts of toxic substances found in our environment, including carcinogens, are stored in fat cells. Because the body uses fat to hold toxins thereby protecting delicate organs, we often find it hard to lose weight. Ironically, fat is our friend when it comes to toxins. It protects us from all the acidic and toxic waste that endangers our organs. But when we remove this mess through detoxing, our bodies no longer need this protection, so they can begin to let go of the extra fat. We suddenly notice that our clothes fit better and we feel lighter and happier, while fat just seems to be melting away.

Juicing and Fasting: The Best Ways to Begin Detoxing

As you prepare to fast and detox, your first step is to add fresh vegetable juices that will help you transition to a healthier diet. The juices will build your body's nutritional reserves and strengthen your immune system. They'll begin to gently detox your body because they are rich in antioxidants that bind to toxins and carry them out of your system. And they prepare your body for more intense cleansing in the form of short juice fasts and detox plans.

Juicing can be fun and easy and the health results are astounding. In chapter two, I'll show you how to incorporate juicing into your busy lifestyle and make sure you look forward to every juice, smoothie, or cold soup you make. And I'll tell you which juicers are best and why. You can learn how to prepare juices quickly and easily and make delicious, nutritious juice.

The recipes in this book use very little fruit juice. Instead I focus on alkaline juicing, which means primarily vegetable juices and raw, blended vegetable soups and smoothies. I show you how to make the juices and soups taste great with additions like lemon or lime, gingerroot, or a little low-sugar fruit such as a green apple, but without the taste of sweeter fruit, while you retrain your taste buds for a whole new juicing experience. Because vegetable juices are alkalizing, they help the body flush away accumulated acidic, toxic waste and enable it to reach a better pH balance so it can cleanse, heal, and get rid of excess weight and cellulite. Almost all toxins are acidic, which is the opposite of alkaline, so drinking lots of vegetable juice, especially plenty of green juices, helps to counteract this acidity.

Most juice books, including my first juice book, *Juicing for Life*, use too much fruit juice, which contains too much sugar. Fruit contains a lot of natural sugar, which is fine when combined with insoluble and soluble fiber. (Fiber slows down sugar absorption.) But when fruit is juiced, the insoluble fiber is removed, and the fruit sugar is easily absorbed. That's why I recommend that you eat your fruit as a general rule, with the exception of low-sugar fruit such as lemon, lime, grapefruit, berries, and green apple, and juice and eat your vegetables.

And for an additional health boost, I advocate adding a short juice fast for one or two days as a great way to jump-start your health or weight loss. It will give your digestive system a rest so it can process and eliminate food and waste that have accumulated over time. Juices are easy to digest and provide concentrated nutrition for energy, plus plenty of vitamins, minerals, enzymes, phytochemicals, and antioxidants. No matter what else you're doing, adding short vegetable-juice fasts occasionally into your diet will help you feel healthier and more energetic right away.

Take the First Steps to a Healthy Lifestyle

The very first step in a healthy lifestyle is choosing the best food and beverages. And once you've finished the detox programs, you can maintain the ground you've gained by continuing with a diet that is based on health-building fresh juices, raw foods (50 to 75 percent of your diet), and whole, organic foods.

Most people find that once they've tried my juice recipes, and completed some of the detox programs, their tastes actually change. The old, unhealthy foods they once loved no longer taste as good. They find themselves craving fresh vegetables, juices, and big green salads instead of sugary snacks or salty chips. They might enjoy an occasional meal of their old fare or a few fattening favorites, but for the most part, they want to eat foods that are fresh, whole, and natural. Once you've made some healthy changes, you should no longer crave the things that have been undermining your health and making you feel less vibrant and well.

Following are the basic components of a healthy lifestyle:

Basics of an Alkaline Diet: Why It Matters

The tissues and organs of our bodies do best if they are sustained at a more alkaline rather than an acidic pH environment. The term "pH" refers to the level of acidity and alkalinity in any environment. Battery acid is an example of a strong acid. Lye, or sodium hydroxide, is an example of a strongly alkaline substance. Water, specifically distilled water, is neutral. The pH scale goes from one to fourteen, with one being most acid, seven being neutral, and fourteen being most alkaline, or basic. Biological systems like the human body must maintain a balance in the mid ranges of this pH scale — between 4.0 and 9.5. Most systems, with the exception of parts of our digestive tract, function best if they are slightly alkaline; for example, saliva should be between 6.5 and 7.5 and urine should be about 7. (You can purchase pH testing strips at your pharmacy and find out just how balanced your system is.)

The typical American diet consists of an abundance of foods that create high levels of acidity in the body once they are metabolized or broken down during digestion. Foods that are broken down to acidic residue are meats, poultry, cheese and other dairy products, fried foods, sugar of all kinds, refined flour products including pastas and breads, soft drinks, coffee, tea, beer, wine, liquor, some fruits, and all junk food. Foods that are alkaline are vegetables, vegetable juices, good oils like coconut oil and olive oil, some nuts, and most legumes.

If most of the food we eat metabolizes into an alkaline ash, it nourishes and strengthens the body and gives

Acid Versus Alkaline Foods

ACID	ALKALINE
• Meats and animal products	• Vegetables
• Dairy products	• Vegetable juices
• Fried foods	• Good oils (coconut oil and olive oil)
• Sugar	• Nuts and seeds
• Grains (bread and pasta)	• Most legumes
• Most fruit	• Alkaline water
• Fast foods and junk food	• Some fruit
• Coffee, tea, soda, and alcohol	

us plenty of energy. On the other hand, if the majority of our food is metabolized into an acidic residue, that is toxic and leads to stress on our delicate organs and tissues. Other factors also contribute to acidity, such as chemical and environmental pollutants, free radicals, and electromagnetic fields, as well as negative thoughts and emotions like fear, worry, anger, and anxiety.

If our cells, tissues, and organs are fed with acidic fluids (due to poor lifestyle choices), they can become inflamed, which can lead to disease. Our blood is especially sensitive to pH changes. It must maintain a level that is slightly alkaline, between 7.35 and 7.45. It's a lot like the body's temperature—too high or too low and we can die; slightly off and we feel sick. In the same way, if the blood becomes too acidic or too basic, we feel sick; if it's way off, we can be in a perilous situation.

To rectify imbalances and reduce acid levels, which

is the imbalance most of us deal with, the body attempts to neutralize acids by dumping alkaline buffers into the bloodstream. The principal buffers that react as neutralizers are calcium phosphate and calcium carbonate, and when they are not present from dietary supply, they're taken from our bones. This may account for why so many women, and even older men, are experiencing osteopenia or osteoporosis. If we are overconsuming acidic foods, our bones become weak and porous. Also, in an acidic environment, we can easily develop painful joints and arthritis, even joint deterioration as in osteoarthritis and degenerative hip joint disease. Our organs and other tissues suffer from inflammation caused by the acidity and shortage of minerals to help neutralize it. An overly acidic body is also a toxic body. Microorganisms like bacteria, viruses, and yeast thrive in an acidic medium as do cancer cells, but they do not thrive in an alkaline environment.

Too much acidity also can cause us to gain weight or prevent us from losing weight. The body tends to store acid in fat cells and hang on to the fat to keep the acidity from doing more damage in other areas of the body. Often, when people bring their bodies into a healthy pH balance, the weight seems to just melt off.

You can best maintain a proper pH by balancing your diet with 50 to 75 percent alkaline foods and juices, along with pure water, exercise, and positive thoughts and emotions. You can still enjoy some of your favorite acidic foods if you make them no more than 25 to 30 percent of your diet.

Good Fats and Oils

It's essential in any healthy dietary program to include plenty of good fats and oils. Many people still think that a low-fat diet is the only way to stay slim and maintain health, but current research has shown that a low-fat diet is unhealthy and points to the importance of providing plenty of essential fatty acids.

For several decades we have been inundated with advertising that promotes vegetable oils like safflower, sunflower, soy, corn, and canola oil. However, these oils are all comprised of long-chain fatty acids (LCTs), which contribute to weight gain because the body tends to store them, rather than burn them. They have also been implicated as contributing to heart disease and other health problems because they oxidize easily (meaning they react with oxygen, for example, and form an oxide). When heated, vegetable oils oxidize and can cause free radical damage; at high heat they form trans fats that generate even more free radicals that cause myriad health problems including heart disease. Once a free-radical reaction is started it can create a chain reaction, which produces more free radicals and can ultimately damage thousands of molecules.

One of the classic signs of old age is the appearance of brown, frecklelike spots known as liver spots. They are signs of free radical deterioration in the lipids (fats) in our skin, thus the name *lipo*fuscin. Oxidation of poly-unsaturated fats and protein by free radical activity in the skin is recognized as one of the major causes of liver spots, along with liver congestion and toxicity. Liver spots don't ordinarily cause physical discomfort, but they do affect our appearance and that can cause emotional discontent. They are a result of internal reactions that can undermine our health. Because cells cannot dispose of the lipofuscin pigment, it gradually accumulates within many cells of the body as we age. Once lipofuscin pigment develops, it tends to stick around for life, but you can prevent further oxidation, and perhaps even reduce the spots you already have, by using the right kind of oils in your diet and on your skin.

I recommend virgin coconut oil and extra-virgin olive oil as the best oils for food preparation and cosmetic use. Coconut oil is made up of primarily medium-chain triglycerides (MCTs). The liver especially likes to burn the MCTs in coconut oil, which means this oil will help you lose weight. MCTs act more like kindling in a fire rather than a big log. Other oils, made up of long-chain triglycerides (LCTs) contribute to weight gain because the body tends to store them rather than burn them. They are also easily oxidized, as already discussed. Take a look at our book *The Coconut Diet* for the Coconut Diet Weight Loss Program that has helped thousands of people lose weight and feel healthier. It offers a full discussion of the benefits of coconut oil and how it compares to other oils, along with information on how to use it in more than seventy delicious recipes.

Olive oil is heart healthy and part of the Mediterranean diet. Olive oil is called *virgin* if it is extracted by means of pressure from millstones. The first pressing is the most flavorful and has the least acidity; it's called extra virgin. The first cold pressing also has the highest amount of fatty acids and polyphenols (antioxidants). Olive oils from the Mediterranean, and particularly Spain, are the highest in antioxidants. The very best choice is extra-virgin, cold-pressed olive oil that is organically grown in the Mediterranean.

Water and the Importance of Hydrating

Our bodies are over 70 percent water, so we need to continually drink purified water to keep properly hydrated. Water is vital to health because it helps flush waste through the system. If you're dehydrated, you can become constipated, acidic, and fatigued. We depend on water for our very existence, yet many people simply do not drink enough, or enough of the right type of water. Fortunately it has become somewhat fashionable to carry water bottles wherever we go, and the educated public is beginning to understand the importance of drinking water. Still, if you ask the average person how much water they drink, they'll probably tell you one or two pint bottles a day. But some people say they don't even like water and refuse to drink it. At least eight to ten eight-ounce glasses of water a day (two to two and a half quarts) is recommended for good health. Three to four quarts a day is optimum if you are detoxing, are a large person, or are very active.

Water increases endurance and energy, aids digestion, regulates body temperature, and facilitates muscular and nervous system activity. Our bodies are designed to deliver essential nutrients, oxygen, hormones, and antibodies into our cells through an aqueous medium. When the body is properly hydrated, it's then able to deliver nutrients and remove toxic waste products that have been accumulating over time.

The water from most kitchen taps is generally not good for drinking. As it travels through the many miles of pipe (many of them in our cities are very old and some are deteriorating) and earth, it picks up thousands of microscopic impurities like pesticides, industrial chemicals, heavy metals, parasites, and other toxins. Most city tap water has added chemicals like chlorine and fluoride, which are also harmful to our bodies. Therefore, it's vitally important that we drink the purest water possible.

Filter Your Water

Most tap water in the United States contains fluoride, a toxic industrial chemical that has been widely promoted as being healthy for the public. In reality, however, fluoride is a poison that may harm your health. Did you know?

- The Canadian Dental Association advises that fluoride is harmful to the development of children's teeth.
- Sodium fluoride is used in rat poison.
- Most of the fluoride (fluosilicic acid) used to fluoridate U.S. water systems comes from the fertilizer industry and may contain trace amounts of various heavy metals such as lead, mercury, and arsenic.
- The only states where less than 25 percent of the tap water is fluoridated are Hawaii, Oregon, Utah, Montana, and New Jersey.

When it comes to purified water, there are several options: distillers, sediment filters, activated carbon filters, kinetic degradation fluxion (KDF) filters, and reverse osmosis. There are water filtration systems that also ionize the water, thus enabling you to set the controls to produce alkaline water, which is a huge plus in keeping your system in alkaline balance.

Whatever you do, avoid bottled water in #7 plastic bottles as much as possible. A number is required on all plastic so you can determine what kind of plastic is used, and #7 is used for almost all plastic water bottles, including the five-gallon bottles for home and office coolers. This plastic used for bottles and many plastic food containers includes phthalates, which are compounds used in inks, adhesives, vinyl floor tiles, and paints.

They make plastic more flexible, but they're troublesome because they leach into the water or food being stored. They have the potential to cause male offspring to be more feminine and develop small or abnormal reproductive organs, and are associated with early puberty in girls and miscarriages in women. Women who are pregnant or planning on getting pregnant should especially avoid water from #7 plastic bottles and #7 plastic food containers. (Look for the number imprinted on the container or bottle, usually on the bottom.)

You can opt for safer choices for water bottles and food and beverage storage, which includes polypropylene (#5 PP), high-density polyethylene (#2 HDPE), and low-density polyethylene (#4 LDPE). No evidence has been found to suggest that these plastics leach toxic materials. For transporting water, you can purchase nontoxic water bottles that don't leach phthalates or aluminum, and don't harbor bacteria. (Go to your health food store or online and you'll find many Web sites that sell nontoxic water bottles.)

Dangerous Chemical Found in Plastic

According to a statement by several dozen scientists, as well as reports from federal health agencies, an estrogen-like compound widely used in plastic products is thought to be causing serious reproductive disorders. The compound is bisphenol A (BPA), and is one of the most-produced chemicals in the world. Almost everyone has traces of it in their bodies. A new study by the National Institutes of Health found that newborn animals exposed to BPA suffered from uterine damage. The damage could indicate that this chemical causes reproductive disorders in women ranging from fibroids to endometriosis to cancer.

After reviewing nearly seven hundred studies, scientists concluded that people are exposed to levels of BPA in excess of those that have harmed lab animals. Among the most vulnerable are infants and fetuses that are still developing. BPA is used to make hard plastic that's used in numerous products including:

- Polycarbonate plastic baby bottles
- Large water-cooler containers and sports bottles
- Microwave-oven dishes
- Canned-food liners
- Some dental sealants for children

Problems associated with even small amounts of BPA include

- Structural damage to the brain
- Hyperactivity
- Abnormal sexual behavior
- Increased fat formation and risk of obesity
- Early puberty and disrupted reproductive cycles

10 Tips to Reduce Your Exposure to BPA

1. Use only glass baby bottles and dishes for your baby
2. Give your baby natural fabric toys instead of plastic ones
3. Store your food and beverages in glass—not plastic containers
4. Avoid using a microwave as much as possible, but if you do, don't microwave food in a plastic container
5. Completely avoid canned foods and drinks
6. Avoid using plastic wrap (and never microwave anything covered in it)
7. Get rid of plastic dishes, glasses, and cups, and replace them with glass
8. If you opt to use plastic kitchenware, at least get rid of the older, scratched-up varieties, avoid putting them in the dishwasher, and don't wash them with harsh detergents, as these things can cause more chemicals to leach into your food. In the event that you do opt to use plastic containers for your food, be sure to avoid those marked on the bottom with the recycling label #7, as these varieties may contain BPA
9. Avoid using bottled water; filter your own instead
10. Before allowing a dental sealant to be applied to your teeth or to your children's, ask your dentist to verify that it does not contain BPA

The Value of Eating Whole Foods

Whole foods are foods that are unprocessed and unrefined, or processed and refined as little as possible before being consumed. Modern food processing strips away nutrients and fiber, and often forms harmful chemicals in the process. These alien food substances are difficult for the body to metabolize.

Often confused with organically grown food, whole foods aren't necessarily organic, nor are organic foods necessarily whole, but organic and whole are the most desirable foods to choose. Because of the lack of preservatives, many whole foods have a short shelf life, but they also have more life-giving nutrients and fewer toxins than processed food. This makes them very desirable when it comes to health.

Examples of whole foods include unpolished grains, unprocessed fruits and vegetables, and unpasteurized milk. The farther away we get from the original food, the less whole it is, such as instant potatoes versus whole potatoes, pressed turkey versus whole turkey, or margarine versus butter or the seeds and vegetables it's made from.

Why It's Important to Eat Raw Foods

It is preferable to eat 50 to 75 percent of our whole foods raw to obtain the maximum nutritional and health-related benefits. Scientific evidence shows that raw foods have significant long-term health benefits. For example, an article published in the *Journal of Nutrition* (April 1992) shows that raw vegan diets significantly decreased LDL cholesterol and triglycerides. Other research shows that shifting from a conventional diet to predominantly foods that are uncooked can result in a decrease in bacterial enzymes and certain toxic products in the body.

So what does heat do to our food? Chemical changes take place to individual nutrients as excessive heat is applied. Excessive heat breaks down vitamins, enzymes, and amino acids and produces undesirable cross-linkages in proteins, particularly in meat. When food is heated above 118 degrees Fahrenheit for three minutes or longer, deleterious changes begin, and progressively cause increased nutritional damage as higher temperatures are applied over longer periods of time. For example, proteins coagulate because high temperatures denature protein molecular structure, leading to deficiency of some essential amino acids. (However, meat, poultry, and fish must be thoroughly cooked at 325 degrees Fahrenheit to 350 degrees Fahrenheit.) Carbohydrates caramelize. And fats oxidize and generate numerous carcinogens including acrolein, nitrosamines, hydrocarbons, and benzopyrene (one of the most potent cancer-causing agents known). Many vitamins are destroyed and most of the enzymes are damaged. Further, the body must produce more enzymes to help digest cooked food, which drains energy needed to maintain and repair tissue and organ systems. Also pesticides can restructure into even more toxic compounds, and free radicals are produced.

Is Microwaving Food Harmful?

The following is a summary of a 1976 Russian investigation published by the Atlantis Raising Educational Center in Portland, Oregon. The investigators found that carcinogens were formed in virtually all foods tested. No test food was subjected to more microwaving than necessary to insure sanitary ingestion. Here's a summary of some of the results:

- Microwaving prepared meats sufficiently to insure sanitary ingestion caused formation of d-Nitrosodienthanolamines, a well-known carcinogen.
- Microwaving milk and cereal grains converted certain amino acids into carcinogens.
- Thawing frozen fruits converted their glucoside- and galactoside-containing fractions into carcinogenic substances.
- Short exposure of raw, cooked, or frozen vegetables converted a portion of their plant alkaloids into carcinogens.
- Free radicals were formed in microwaved root vegetables.
- Ingestion of microwaved foods caused a higher percentage of cancerous cells in blood.
- Due to chemical alterations within food substances, malfunctions occurred in the lymphatic system, causing degeneration of the immune system's capacity to protect itself against cancerous growth.

There are many things you can do to preserve your food, such as dehydrating things like crackers, onions, tomatoes, and even kale and Swiss chard at 118 degrees Fahrenheit or below (considered raw food); they are healthful and delicious! (See Resources Guide for dehydrator recommendations.) And you can gently warm vegetable foods (not animal products), keeping the temperature at 118 degrees Fahrenheit or below, which helps to preserve nutrient content.

The reasons why raw foods are so life-giving haven't been thoroughly researched, but the experience is unmistakable. Eating more raw organic food is one of the best ways to secure your health; it builds your immune system and prevents disease. Finding ways to get more raw foods into your diet, such as juicing every day, is one of the keys to vibrant health.

Making Wise Food Choices

Make these food choices a major part of your diet:

- Whole, unprocessed food
- Organically grown food
- Fresh vegetables
- Raw nuts and seeds
- Whole grains
- Legumes (beans, lentils, split peas)
- Whole low-sugar fruit
- Free-range poultry (in small amounts)
- Grass-fed beef (in small amounts)
- Kosher and free-range meats (in small amounts)
- Organic, free-range eggs
- Plenty of alkaline foods
- Good fats and oils (virgin coconut oil and extra-virgin olive oil)
- Plenty of purified water, stored in nontoxic water bottles
- Minimize or avoid stimulants such as coffee and tea (herbal is fine) and alcohol

---

Exercise

Exercise is essential for a strong body and vibrant health. And it keeps us trim and fit so we look great and have plenty of energy for daily work and recreation. Exercise physiologists tell us that even short periods of exercise over time will provide enormous benefits. We will not only look and feel better; we will be nourished and strengthened — inside and out.

Daily exercise or movement of some kind is also necessary for effective internal function of our bodies. It is especially crucial during the detoxing process because the movement carries waste products out of our system and strengthens the immune system. Regular movement also keeps the heart and cardiovascular system strong, enables the body to properly metabolize nutrients, and builds new proteins and hormones. It also helps us sleep better at night, a big plus for the cleansing, healing process.

Emotional and Spiritual Health

Our lives are often harried and stressful. We're under pressure to do more than we have time or energy to accomplish. Negative, angry, critical, or unforgiving thoughts about ourselves and others can wreak havoc on our nervous, cardiovascular, and endocrine systems, which then affects every organ and tissue in our body, often translating into myriad health problems.

Even if you are eating well and exercising regularly, negative thoughts and emotions can bring about a cascading response from the endocrine system, which releases hormones like adrenaline and cortisol that lead to fight-or-flight reactions. Constant overstimulation and exposure to these stress hormones weakens our immune system and eventually leads to diseases and biological disorders. Stress also damages the liver, which is the principal organ of detoxification in the body; it is also quite sensitive to anger. And it can weaken the kidneys, which are particularly sensitive to fear, and the lungs, which are very sensitive to grief. While our bodies are healing and we are cleansing, we should care for and nurture our souls. (See chapter eight for an extensive discussion of thoughts and emotions as they relate to detoxing and to health.)

A Pep Talk for the Juicing, Fasting, and Detox Programs

Some days we're just too busy or stressed out to stay on a strict program, so don't try to be perfect all the time, just do the best you can. And remember, it's still better to do *something* good for yourself rather than lapse into totally unhealthy patterns. Ask yourself: "Is this going to make me feel better and build my health, or is it going to make me feel worse and undermine my hard work?" If you're mad at yourself about a little indulgence or about getting off a cleanse program, you may slip back into some old, unhealthy patterns and just decide to blow it completely. Instead, love and forgive yourself for not being perfect. Get a little exercise, relax, take a few deep breaths, pick up a good book, pray or meditate, spend time with friends and family, and get back in the rhythm of a healthy life. No one's perfect, but you want to feel good and care for the wonderful body you've been given so you'll have energy for work, pleasure, and enjoying your friends and family. Tell yourself that you can do it. You're a strong person who deserves to experience vibrant health.

Summary of The Secrets of Vibrant Health

- Reduce environmental toxins.
- Make wise food choices.
- Increase exercise.
- Find emotional, mental, and spiritual balance.

CHAPTER TWO

Juicing for Life

Recently, someone asked me if they couldn't just drink V8 juice and eat more salads and get the same effect as juicing fresh produce. First, most of us just can't seem to eat enough fresh vegetables each day to even reach the minimum number of servings suggested for good health. And processed juice—canned, bottled, or frozen—has had a lot of nutrients destroyed in the processing, so they fall short when it comes to revitalizing the body. But probably the most compelling reason to juice is that fresh juice provides an excellent way for us to absorb vitamins and minerals, which is even superior to eating whole vegetables, because juicing releases these nutrients in a highly absorbable form. So as you embark on your journey to vibrant health, eat whole foods—at least 50 to

75 percent of them should be raw. Drink plenty of water. And juice a lot of vegetables most days of the week.

If you're wondering how you can possibly fit juicing into a schedule that is so busy you can barely get everything done in a day, I'll show you how to make it work. Some people say they're intimidated by the whole prospect of juicing, imagining it to be a daunting, messy, and time-consuming process. Others think it's so difficult that only professionals can do it right, so they never even get started. One lady told me she drove around with a juicer in the trunk of her car for two months before she had the courage to even take it inside her house. If you're among those who are confused or intimidated, I'll help you. There are dozens of tips on how to choose and use a juicer in the pages that follow. You'll be "juicing it up" in no time. And if you're still a bit confused, just go to my Web site for more information; then, if you still need extra help, contact me. I'll get you through the process (see Resources Guide).

The good news is that there are many ways to make juicing quick, easy, and a regular part of your life. When you've finished this chapter, you'll see that even a beginner can have a juicer up and running in a short time. The latest juicers are designed for busy people because the manufacturers have figured out that most people won't use them unless they're easy to operate and clean. Some of the newest machines are very fast. I've timed myself and found that I can make the morning juice for my husband and myself in about ten minutes from start to finish, which includes cleanup. There are juicers with superwide feeding tubes at the top so you don't have to cut produce up into little pieces. The best ones are designed to expel the pulp into a container that you can line with a free baggie from the grocery store produce section. That way, you can just dump the whole thing in the trash or the compost pile when you're done and you don't have to wash the pulp catcher. Plus, most of the newer-model juicers are easier than ever to clean because they have only a few parts to wash and most of those are dishwasher safe.

There are also steps you can take in advance to save time. For example, you can wash and prepare your produce the night before or perhaps on the weekend to make juicing in the morning even faster. You can place your washed produce in airtight containers, Ziploc bags, or the new green bags that keep produce fresh longer. That way you can grab a handful of each of your favorite veggies with a bit of low-sugar fruit, toss them in the juicer, and be done juicing in a matter of minutes. (You can also make your juice the night before and store it in an airtight container.) Then simply rinse off the juicer parts and place them in the upper rack of your dishwasher. It's really that easy. Either drink the juice right away or store it in an airtight container like a thermos and be off for the day! And you can make extra juice for later. It's great to have some freshly made juice for a midmorning break at work or with lunch.

It's possible — and easy — to juice up more produce in one glass than many people will eat in a day — maybe even more than you'd put in a big main-course salad. For example, on most mornings, I juice one very large cucumber, two to four carrots, a handful of parsley, two stalks of celery, a two-inch piece of gingerroot, and half a lemon. (This serves two and that's just our starting juice for the day.)

Once you realize how healthy and energizing it is to drink fresh juice each day, and how great you feel, I think you'll be motivated to find a way to juice up your favorite produce on a regular basis. Whether you're a busy executive, a career mom or dad, or someone who's just always on the go, juicing will give you the energy and vitality to accomplish more and feel great while you're doing it. And you don't want to wait until you're sick, like I did, to start a health-building program. Juicing is the best fast food in the world — it provides quick energy that lasts throughout the day and will put you on the fast track to health. You'll find you just aren't as hungry so it's easier to maintain your weight. When you drink this life-giving nutrition in a glass, you're sowing great seeds of health that will serve you for years to come.

Fresh Juice or Liquid Candy

Fresh juice prepared at home in your juicer is one of the healthiest alternatives to other popular beverages like soft drinks, which contain ten teaspoons of sugar. But whether they're sugar sweetened or artificially sweetened diet sodas, soft drinks contribute to obesity and a host of other health problems. That's because the massive amount of sugar they contain causes an insulin burst that turns the sugar into fat. A recent study showed that those who drink two to three regular soft drinks a day have a 35 percent greater chance of being overweight. Diet sodas are even more likely to pack on the pounds. Surprisingly, 55 percent of the people who drank two to three diet sodas per day were shown to be overweight. Diet sodas and other diet products contain artificial sweeteners that overexcite the nervous system, causing people to want more and more sweet foods. Studies showed that those who drank the most artificially sweetened beverages gained the most weight. Artificial sweeteners, such as aspartame, have been associated with brain tumors. Sucralose (Splenda) has been associated with thymus gland shrinkage.

Components of a Can of Soda

- **Phosphoric acid** can interfere with the body's ability to use calcium, leading to osteoporosis or softening of the teeth and bones. It also neutralizes hydrochloric acid in your stomach, which can interfere with digestion, making it difficult to utilize nutrients.
- **Sugar** increases insulin levels, which can lead to high blood pressure, high cholesterol, heart disease, diabetes, weight gain, premature aging, and many more negative side effects.
- **Aspartame** is used as a sugar substitute in diet soda. There are numerous side effects associated with aspartame consumption including brain tumors, birth defects, diabetes, emotional disorders, and epilepsy and seizures.
- **Caffeine** in drinks causes jitters, insomnia, high blood pressure, irregular heartbeat, elevated blood cholesterol levels, vitamin and mineral depletion, breast lumps, and birth defects.
- **Tap water** is the main ingredient in bottled soft drinks. It can carry numerous chemicals including chlorine, trihalomethanes, lead, cadmium, and various organic pollutants.

Sodas also contribute to toxicity. They contain artificial colorings, especially Yellow dye No. 5, which has been shown to promote attention-deficit

(Continued)

hyperactivity disorder (ADHD) in some children. Yellow dye No. 5 also causes hives, asthma, and other allergic reactions in a small number of individuals. The chemicals in sodas break down into even more toxic by-products once ingested, taxing the liver and leading to symptoms such as headaches, depression, lethargy, certain autoimmune disorders, and low thyroid function. Also, they can lead to low blood sugar, diabetes, and cravings for more sweet carbohydrates. Consumption of soft drinks may also increase the risk of osteoporosis because phosphorus, a common ingredient in soda, has been shown to deplete bones of calcium.

So when you're on the go, take fresh juice in a thermos for a healthy pick-me-up. There are also unsweetened waters with flavors such as cranberry-orange, pear, pomegranate-tangerine, and raspberry-lime. These are much healthier choices than the "liquid candy" people are downing.

Psychologists tell us it takes about twenty-one days to develop a new habit, and those twenty-one days of juicing will propel you into a whole new level of health. To help motivate you, the next section will give you an overview of the many ways juicing can build your health and energize every cell in your body. You'll also find nutritional information about what vegetable juice contains, so you'll know more about what it's doing for you. Once you see all the benefits, you just may be sold on juicing for the rest of your life.

Why Drink Juice?

Fresh juice contains an abundance of nutrients that will energize your body, build your health, and help you fight disease. Juice provides water, easily absorbed amino acids and carbohydrates, plus a virtual cornucopia of vitamins, minerals, enzymes, antioxidants, phytonutrients, and soluble fiber. Scientists are now showing that the phytonutrients found in plants may be even more important for our health than vitamins and minerals. Without all these life-giving substances, found principally in vegetables and fruit, our immune systems weaken and we become subject to various disturbances, which can lead to feeling sick and tired most of the time and to illness and disease.

Forget the "5 a day"! The latest nutritional guidelines show that we need between nine and thirteen servings of vegetables and fruit per day to stay healthy, depending on age and activity level, with an emphasis on dark green leafy vegetables and red and yellow vegetables and fruit. It was hard enough to get enough to get even five of these life-giving foods in our diet each and every day. Juicing is about the only way many of us can get more. The following equals one serving: half a cup of raw or cooked vegetables, three-quarters cup of vegetable juice, and one cup of raw leafy vegetables. So if you're going for the minimum of nine servings daily, you'll need something like one to two cups green leafy vegetables (that's about one salad) and four cups fruits and vegetables. That's not easy to do most days. Juicing can really help you fill in the gaps. When you juice a lot of veggies, eat a piece or two of fruit, have a big salad and a steamed vegetable, you'll reach the recommended goal.

There's another great benefit. Because fresh juice is loaded with antioxidants that bind to toxins and carry them out of the body so they don't damage your cells, it offers a gentle way to begin detoxifying your system. Your digestive system doesn't have to expend a lot of energy to break down juice. Therefore, it can use the energy to detoxify your body, make repairs, and build your health. Scientists are continuing to discover how various nutrients found in fresh juice build your immune system, help prevent disease, and heal specific ailments. See the box below regarding the latest research on the healing benefits of vegetables, keeping in mind that juice made from these foods makes the nutrients in them highly available to fight off diseases and build immunity.

Scientific Research and the Healing Benefits of Vegetables and Fruit

Following are various diseases science has shown can be helped with a diet rich in vegetables and fruit.

Cardiovascular Disease

A diet rich in vegetables and fruit has been found to lower the risk of heart disease and stroke. The most comprehensive research study to date was done by the Harvard School of Public Health. They followed the health and dietary habits of 110,000 men and women for fourteen years, and found that the higher the average-daily intake of vegetables and fruit, the lower the chances of developing cardiovascular disease. Those who averaged eight or more servings a day were 30 percent less likely to have had a heart attack or stroke than those eating less. Green leafy vegetables such as lettuce, spinach, Swiss chard, mustard greens; cruciferous vegetables such as broccoli, cauliflower, cabbage, Brussels sprouts, bok choy, and kale; and citrus fruit such as oranges, lemons, limes, and grapefruit seem to have the greatest benefit.

Cancer

Scientists have long noted that there is a strong link between eating plenty of vegetables and fruit and protection against certain cancers. The International Agency for Research on Cancer, which is part of the World Health Organization, conducted a huge review of the best research on fruit, vegetables, and cancer. They concluded that consumption of fruit and vegetables helped prevent cancers of the mouth and pharynx, esophagus, stomach, colon-rectum, larynx, lung, ovary, bladder, and kidney. They noted that eating more vegetables will lower the risk of cancers of the esophagus and colon-rectum and possibly reduce the risk of cancers of the mouth, pharynx, stomach, larynx, lung, ovaries, and kidneys.

High Blood Pressure

A study called the DASH (the Dietary Approaches to Stop Hypertension) found that a diet rich in fruit, vegetables, and low-fat dairy products was able to significantly reduce the blood pressure of the subjects by as much as if they had used blood pressure–lowering medications. Because high blood pressure is a risk factor for heart disease and stroke, this is a significant finding.

High Cholesterol

The National Heart, Lung, and Blood Institute's Family Heart Study found that eating more vegetables and fruit will help lower cholesterol. This large study followed over four thousand men and women who ate at least three servings of vegetables and fruit a day. Those with the highest daily consumption (more than four servings a day) had significantly lower levels of LDL (bad cholesterol) than those with lower consumption. The researchers speculated that the participants' higher intake of vegetables and fruit limited how much meat and dairy products they were consuming. Another possibility is that the fiber in vegetables and fruit actually blocks the absorption of cholesterol from food.

(Continued)

Vision Problems

The Age-Related Eye Disease Study (AREDS) showed that a daily supplement of 500 milligrams (mg) of vitamin C, 400 international units (IU) of vitamin E, 15 mg of beta-carotene (often as vitamin A—up to 25,000 IU), 80 mg of zinc (as zinc oxide) and 2 mg of copper (as cupric oxide) reduced the risk of progressing to moderate or severe vision loss by up to 25 percent. Consuming vegetables and fruit, either juiced or whole, provides a host of these nutrients, and reduces the chances of developing cataracts or macular degeneration. The provitamin A in carrots (known as carotenes), a favorite for juicing, promotes good vision. The phytonutrients in blueberries helps improve night vision. And dark green leafy vegetables are especially helpful because they contain two pigments, lutein and zeaxanthin, which attack free radicals before they can damage the eyes. There are many other vegetables and fruit that help prevent these two common eye diseases, which are frequently seen in Americans over the age of sixty-five.

Fresh juice not only contains most of the nutrients found in whole vegetables and fruit, they are also easily digested, thus providing good nutrient absorption. In addition, fresh vegetable juices are very alkalizing, so they are extremely beneficial to assist the body in detoxifying, which enables us to further resist disease, lose weight, and heal our bodies.

I have lectured and taught extensively about juicing. I've heard hundreds of personal testimonies from people who have been healed from numerous ailments ranging from heart disease to arthritis, chronic fatigue syndrome, fibromyalgia, and cancer. I know that incorporating fresh vegetable juices into your diet will assist your body to lose weight, heal, and rejuvenate. The nutrients in fresh juice help repair damaged cells and keep healthy cells strong. Once you remove as many of the sources of toxicity as possible by changing your diet to healthy choices, add fresh vegetable juice, and follow the cleansing programs outlined in the pages that follow, your body can remove irritating substances and restore healthy balance.

Margo's Story

I started juicing because I wanted better health and because I had lots of digestive problems. I had no idea that I'd also get rid of the pain in my left foot, and I could hardly walk before. I've noticed that my eyes are brighter, too.

What About the Fiber?

Fiber is the portion of the plant that moves food through the digestive system. It is generally categorized as either soluble or insoluble. Both types of fiber help to increase bulk, soften stools, and shorten the transit time of food moving through the intestinal tract. Both soluble and insoluble fibers are present in whole plant foods like vegetables, fruit, legumes, and grains. There is only soluble fiber in juice.

Soluble fiber in the form of pectins, gums, and mucilages partially dissolves in water, forming a type of gel; it is not digested. Soluble fiber absorbs digestive bile, which is made from cholesterol. When it's eliminated, it causes more cholesterol to be converted to digestive bile, thereby lowering LDL cholesterol. Soluble fiber also helps sugar be more slowly absorbed, which helps regulate blood sugar and control diabetes. The best vegetable sources of soluble fiber are broccoli, carrots, Brussels sprouts, sweet potatoes, turnips, beets, squash, and pumpkin, all of which can be juiced. Soluble fiber is also found in nuts, legumes, barley, flaxseeds, psyllium husks, and oats and oat bran.

Insoluble fiber is also indigestible, but does not dissolve in water. It absorbs water and serves as a bulking agent as it passes through the digestive system. Insoluble fiber promotes regular bowel movements and prevents constipation, as well as helps to maintain a balanced pH in the intestines. It is important in cleansing because it removes toxic substances that tend to accumulate in the colon. Insoluble fiber is abundant in vegetables like dark green leafy vegetables, green beans, and root vegetable skins, along with fruit skins and whole grains like oats and wheat, corn bran, seeds, and nuts.

In the past it was thought that a significant amount of nutrients remained in the fiber of fruits and vegetables after juicing, but that theory has been disproved. The Department of Agriculture analyzed twelve fruits and found that 90 percent of the antioxidant activity was in the juice rather than the fiber.

It was also thought that juice had no fiber. Juicing got a bad rap in the early nineties and lingers on to this day. The media focused on the lack of fiber in juice. But that assertion was simply not true; only the insoluble fiber is removed in the juicing process, and it's loaded with soluble fiber, which is excellent for the intestinal tract. A new study has disproved the idea that even the removal of the insoluble fiber makes fresh juice inferior. A 2006 review of eleven studies conducted by British researchers challenged the belief that fresh juices are not as beneficial as whole vegetables and fruit because they contain less fiber. The study, published in the *International Journal of Food Sciences and Nutrition*, found that "Cancer and cardiovascular benefits may be more attributable to antioxidants rather than fibre." The researchers concluded that "[the theory that] pure fruit and vegetable juices are nutritionally inferior to [whole] fruit and vegetables, in relation to chronic disease risk reduction, is not justified."

The recommended fiber intake for adults is between 20 and 35 grams per day, but the average American's daily intake of dietary fiber is only around 14 to 15 grams. Increasing vegetable consumption by juicing will significantly add to the daily intake of soluble fiber. In addition to fresh juice, eat more whole vegetables and fruit, include a leafy green salad every day, and eat plenty of nuts, seeds, legumes, and whole grains as part of a well-balanced, high-fiber diet. Also, adding flax fiber, psyllium husks, or other high-fiber bulking agents to your juice is another great way to increase your total fiber intake.

THE COMPONENTS OF JUICE

In addition to fiber, fresh juice contains a wide variety of the nutrients that we need for health and wellness. The following list gives you a quick overview of what you get by adding fresh juice to your diet.

Water. Juice made from fresh produce provides an abundance of water, which is the body's most important nutrient. Water makes up 70 to 75 percent of our total body weight and is involved in every bodily function. Water helps maintain body temperature, metabolizes body fat, generates energy, transports nutrients, and flushes toxins out of the body. It also lubricates joints and cushions delicate tissues and organs. Without adequate water our bodies cannot function properly. Adding juice to your diet provides one of our most important requirements for health — water.

Protein. There are a variety of amino acids found in juice, which are the building blocks of protein. Next to water, protein is the most plentiful component of our bodies. Protein is contained in every cell. It's needed to form structures like hair, skin, eyes, nails, muscles, connective tissue, and organs. It's also required for a host of biochemical processes. The body uses the material of protein digestion, amino acids, to build enzymes, which regulate chemical reactions and hormones.

Although vegetables and fruit contain incomplete protein, the amino acids are easily absorbed. Combining other protein sources, such as beans, lentils, dried peas, whole grains, and some low-fat animal proteins to your diet will supplement the vegetable protein in juice. Animal products like meat, poultry, fish, eggs, and dairy products contain the most complete form of protein. For some people, animal protein can be difficult to digest, and so more vegetable sources are required such as legumes (beans, lentils, split peas), nuts, seeds, and whole grains. Also, keep in mind that large quantities of animal protein can cause acidic by-products.

Carbohydrates. Juice contains an abundance of carbohydrates, which are the energy-producing substances that fuel our bodies. They are made up of simple sugar molecules, which are composed of the elements carbon, hydrogen, and oxygen. Complex carbohydrates, or starches, are basically chains of sugar molecules, often containing hundreds of these molecules. Carbohydrates are formed in plants when they receive energy from the sun and store it in their chemical bonds. The energy contained in these carbohydrate molecules is then released when the body metabolizes the plant food as fuel. The three categories of carbohydrates are simple sugars, complex carbohydrates, and fiber. Because fruit juice has a high concentration of simple sugars, mainly fructose, it is recommended that you use fruit juice sparingly — no more than four ounces per day. Vegetables and fruit contain both soluble and insoluble fiber; juice contains only soluble fiber.

Essential Fatty Acids (EFAs). Juice contains only a small amount of fatty acids. Because we need essential fats for energy production and the formation of nerve cells, cellular membranes, and special hormones like prostaglandins, we need to supplement our diet with EFAs. A great way is to first make some fresh juice, then pour it into your blender and add an avocado, some ground flaxseeds (a good source of omega-3 fatty acids), and blend; this makes a satisfying and nourishing vegetable smoothie. You'll also need to supplement your diet with fish oil, krill oil, cod liver oil, or flax oil for ample omega-3 fatty acids. And you could include some omega-3–rich cold-water fish such as wild-caught salmon (avoid farm raised). Your hair, skin, joints, and heart will be happy!

Vitamins. Fresh juice is sometimes called "liquid vitamins" because it supplies so many of these vital nutrients. Vitamins are the organic nutrients required in small amounts to maintain growth and normal metabolism. Most vitamins serve as coenzymes and are part of many reactions in the body. The majority of vitamins can't be synthesized; they must be ingested. Fresh vegetable and fruit juices are excellent sources of water-soluble vitamins, principally many of the B complex vitamins (except B12, which is found in animal products), vitamin C, and the phytochemical, flavonoids. Fresh juice also contains some of the fat-soluble vitamins, notably carotenes (known as provitamin A), vitamin E, and vitamin K.

Minerals. A wide array of minerals is found in fresh juice. The major minerals in our bodies are calcium, chloride, magnesium, phosphorus, potassium, sodium, and sulfur. Trace minerals, which are required in very small amounts, include boron, chromium, cobalt, copper, fluoride, manganese, molybdenum, nickel, selenium, vanadium, and zinc. Our bodies need minerals for many functions such as bone and blood formation and to maintain the proper functioning of the cells. Along with vitamins, minerals are required for enzymes to function, particularly in the production of energy. Minerals are inorganic elements that plants absorb from the soil and then incorporate into their tissues by combining with organic molecules. These organic plant molecules can then be ingested in a usable form that will provide us with the minerals we need to be healthy.

Enzymes. Biochemical processes can't take place in the body without the presence of enzymes. They are necessary for thousands of processes, such as metabolism, energy production, and the building and repair of cells.

Enzymes have been called the "workforce" of the body, and without them, our cells would not survive. Fresh juice is loaded with enzymes because it's made from raw, live produce. Heating, as happens in cooking, blanching, pasteurization, or canning, destroys them. When we drink juice made from fresh vegetables and fruit we are supplying our body with an abundance of the enzymes it needs to digest the food, which spares our organs from working overtime to supply enzymes. This allows the body's energy to be shifted from digestion to other functions such as repair and detoxification, which is one reason why people who regularly drink fresh juice usually notice that their energy levels increase.

Phytochemicals. Known as "plant chemicals," phytochemicals, also called phytonutrients, are produced by plants to protect them from disease, injury, and pollution. They also give plants their color, odor, and flavor. There are tens of thousands of phytochemicals in the vegetables and fruit we eat. For example, the average tomato may contain up to ten thousand different types of these nutrients. Phytochemicals are more stable to heat than vitamins and enzymes, so they can withstand cooking. Nevertheless, drinking them in fresh juice provides much more concentration because we usually juice more than we could chew at one time.

Though they may sound like ingredients found in shampoo, phytochemicals such as allyl sulfides, curcumins, ellagic acid, gingerol, indoles, isothiocyanates, sulforaphanes, limonene, lycopene, and monoterpenes can prevent a host of diseases. Research shows that people who eat plenty of vegetables and fruit have the lowest incidence of cancer, particularly stomach, breast, lung, prostate, skin, liver, and pancreas. They've also been shown to help reduce inflammation, lower cholesterol levels, fight viruses, heal ulcers, increase immune function, stimulate detoxification enzymes, and protect DNA from damage. Foods like garlic, onions, ginger, turmeric, strawberries, cruciferous vegetables (broccoli, cabbage, and cauliflower), citrus fruit, tomatoes, berries, and cherries are particularly rich in phytonutrients.

Choosing the Best Juicer

Now that you know a lot about why juicing is good for you, all you need is a good juicer to get started. A juicer and a blender are different. A juicer separates the liquid juice from the pulp. You drink the juice and toss the pulp or compost it. On the other hand, a blender doesn't separate the pulp from the juice. Even the high-speed types like the Vita-Mix simply whirl everything around and mix it up. You generally have to add some liquid like water or juice to get things going. Blenders are great for making smoothies and cold soups with soft produce, but they won't make juice. Blended hard vegetables such as carrots, beets, and stringy veggies like celery turn out quite gritty. If you try to make carrot juice with water and carrots in your blender, you'll have a very fiber-thick, mushy taste like carrot-flavored sawdust. I recommend you use a juicer for vegetable juice.

FEATURES OF A GOOD JUICER

Choosing the right juicer will determine whether you become dedicated to juicing or try it a few times and never juice again. You can spend lots of money on some juicers, and though they may be good quality, many are a hassle to clean. You may save money on a chain store bargain, but it won't do you much good if it sits in your bottom cupboard because it's a big hassle to use. Here's what to look for:

Adequate Horsepower: Choose a juicer that is at least one-third to one-half horsepower (hp). Weak machines with low horsepower ratings must run at extremely high rpm (revolutions per minute). A machine's rpm does not accurately reflect its ability to perform effectively, because rpm is calculated when the juicer is running idle, not while it is juicing. However, when you feed produce into a low-power machine, the rpm will be reduced dramatically, and sometimes the juicer will come to a full stop. I have "killed" some machines on the first carrot I juiced.

Maintains Blade Speed: Look for a machine that

has electronic circuitry that sustains blade speed during juicing.

Doesn't Need Special Tool to Loosen Juicer Blade: There are a few popular machines that require a special tool to get the blade out for washing and to tighten it again. Lose the tool and you can't use your juicer.

Strong Enough for Hard Vegetables: Make sure the machine can juice tough, hard vegetables, such as carrots and beets, as well as delicate greens, such as parsley, lettuce, and herbs.

Doesn't Need Special Citrus Attachment: Make sure you can use the juicer for citrus fruit such as lemons and limes.

Large Feeding Tube: This feature allows you to put whole or large pieces of produce in the juicer, so you don't have to cut everything up into little pieces, which saves significant time and energy.

Ejects Pulp into Receptacle: Choose a juicer that ejects the pulp into a receptacle. This design is far better than one in which all the pulp stays inside the machine, and so has to be scooped out frequently. Juicers that keep the pulp in the center basket rather than ejecting it cannot juice continuously. You'll need to stop the machine often to wash it out. One time saver — you can line the receptacle with a baggie, which eliminates the need for washing. That's one less part to hassle with.

Few Parts to Clean: Look for a juicer with only a few

parts to clean. The more parts a juicer has, and the more complicated the parts are to wash, the longer it will take to clean your juicer and put it back together. The fewer parts to clean, the more likely you'll be to use it daily. Also, make sure the parts are dishwasher safe.

Now it's time to begin juicing. I have plenty of delicious recipes for you in chapter ten and suggestions along the way. So grab your juicer, or go buy one, and get started juicing right away!

Juicing Made Simple

Now that you know all about the best juicers, it's time to begin! If you're a little intimidated or puzzled about how to start, rest assured; it's really quite simple. Just follow these few easy steps and you're on your way.

STEP 1: **Buy enough produce to make the juice you want.** Figure out how much juice you want to make. I recommend at least one to two eight-ounce glasses a day per person, but you'll need more if you're cleansing or doing a juice fast. To make one eight-ounce glass of juice takes about a pound of produce; for example, two or three carrots, half a lemon, one or two stalks celery, and a cucumber. You may want to add green leafy vegetables like spinach, kale, or parsley, which can be strong tasting, so it's always best to mix them with the other mild-tasting vegetables.

STEP 2: **Wash all the produce before juicing.** Washing your produce is something you can do ahead of time. Store it in the refrigerator in glass or plastic containers or green produce bags so it's all ready for later. Most health food stores and many grocery stores have vegetable washes that you can purchase for removing toxins and dirt. (Be aware that washes cannot remove pesticides that are systemic, meaning that they are found throughout the plant.) Or, you can fill your sink or a large container with sea salt and wash the produce in the salt solution. Use a vegetable brush to remove the dirt, even for organic produce.

STEP 3: **Prepare the produce.** Be sure to cut off any parts that are bruised, moldy, or damaged. Peel the following:

- Anything not labeled organic should be peeled, as the pesticides are concentrated in the peel (unfortunately so are the nutrients).
- Lemons and limes don't have to be peeled if they are organic, but many people like to peel them since the skin can be a little bitter.

What to take out and what to leave in:

- **Take out** pits, stones, and hard seeds
- **Leave in** softer seeds
- **Leave on** the stems and leaves of most produce, such

as beet greens and parsley stems, as there's a lot of nutritional value in them; take off hard stems.

◆ **Cut off** carrot greens because they contain toxic substances.

STEP 4: **Start cutting things up.** Cut the vegetables and fruit (primarily that's lemon, lime, or green apple) into sections that will fit your juicer's feed tube. Many of the new juicers have very wide feeding tubes that enable you to put in whole small beets, tomatoes, small apples, small lemons, limes, and large carrots, without cutting them at all. Larger items like cabbage, cauliflower, and so forth obviously need to be cut in smaller pieces. It won't take you long to figure out what works with your juicer.

STEP 5: **Prepare to catch the pulp.** Line the pulp receptacle with a plastic bag; you can use the free ones you get in the grocery store produce section. When you're finished juicing, toss the baggie with the pulp or throw it in your compost pile. Then you won't have to wash out the receptacle — saving you even more time.

STEP 6: **Prepare to catch the juice.** This may seem obvious, but unless your juicer comes with its own container to catch the juice (some do; most don't), you'll need to find a container that is tall enough and wide enough so the juice doesn't end up on the counter. Any container will do, as long as it's the right size.

STEP 7: What to do with produce you can't juice. Avocados don't juice well since they don't contain enough water. Add them to juices like carrot, lemon, and cucumber by combining them in a blender. This makes a delicious satisfying cold soup or smoothie. Bananas won't juice either, but they work well in a smoothie.

STEP 8: Drink your juice! If possible, it's best to drink your juice as soon as it's prepared. Freshly made juice contains the most nutrients; the longer it sits, the more it loses. If you need to make juice ahead of time because you can't juice in the morning or during the day, then store it in an insulated container like a thermos, or another type of airtight, opaque container in the refrigerator. You can store it for up to twenty-four hours. It will still lose some nutrients, but it's far better than anything you can buy already bottled. Many of the nutrients like vitamins, enzymes, and some phytochemicals are affected by light and heat, which causes them to oxidize. As you might guess, if the juice turns brown, that's a sign that it has oxidized and has lost a good share of its nutritional value. Cabbage juice should be consumed as soon as you make it, as it does not store well.

On a personal note: When I had chronic fatigue

syndrome, I would juice in the afternoons, when I had the most energy, and store the juice covered in the refrigerator and drink it for the next twenty-four hours until I juiced my next batch. I got well doing this, so I can assure you that a lot of nutrients remained intact even though refrigerated for up to twenty-four hours.

Choose Organic Produce

The best way to get the healthiest juice possible is to buy organic produce whenever you can. It is even more important when cleansing to avoid ingesting pesticides and other toxic products—the very stuff you're trying to get rid of. Certified organic vegetables and fruit are grown without pesticides, fungicides, herbicides, or chemical fertilizers. And organic farmers don't use genetically modified seeds. Always look for food that is labeled "certified organic." This means the produce has been cultivated according to strict uniform standards that are verified by independent state or private organizations. Certification includes inspection of farms and processing facilities, detailed record keeping, and pesticide testing of soil and water to ensure that growers and handlers are meeting government standards.

Researchers say there is now firm evidence that choosing organic foods helps you avoid toxic pesticides. In 1995 the USDA tested nearly seven thousand conventionally grown fruit and vegetable samples and detected residues of sixty-five different pesticides, with two out of three samples containing pesticide residue.

In recent years, increased awareness among the health-conscious public has made organic foods much easier to find. Many grocery stores now have organic sections and health food stores and natural foods chains have sprung up all across the country. There are organic food co-ops, buying clubs, and organic farmers' markets in nearly every part of the country. The sale of organic foods has become a multibillion-dollar industry. As more people become educated about the wholesale use of pesticides and herbicides and the negative health effects, they are demanding organic food. That's because pesticide residues have been shown to cause numerous long-term health risks, such as cancer and birth defects, and immediate health risks from acute intoxication, such as vomiting, diarrhea, blurred vision, tremors, convulsions, and nerve damage.

Many studies have shown that organically grown vegetables and fruit have been found to have higher concentrations of vitamins and minerals than those that are cultivated inorganically. While organic foods are always the best option in terms of avoiding pesticides, studies also show they are higher in nutrient content. In a 2001 study published in the *Journal of Alternative and Complementary Medicine*, on average, organic produce contained 27 percent more vitamin C, 21 percent more iron, and 29 percent more magnesium than conventional produce, and all twenty-one minerals compared in the study were higher in the organic produce. Additionally, research has shown that organic food contains more secondary metabolites than conventionally grown plants. Secondary metabolites are substances that form part of the plants' immune system, and that helps fight cancer in humans.

Chemical fertilizers can reduce the quality of nutrition. For example, the quality of protein in grains and vegetables is related to the amount of nitrogen in the soil. When there is a lot of nitrogen present, plants increase protein production and decrease carbohydrate synthesis. When the metabolic protein requirements are satisfied, the remaining protein produced is stored in a form that contains fewer essential amino acids. The result of high levels of nitrogen, as found in conventional chemical fertilizers, is an increase in the amount of protein but a reduction in its quality. Organically managed soils release nitrogen in smaller amounts over a longer time than conventional fertilizers. As a result, the quality of protein from organic crops is better in terms of human nutrition.

If you'd like to stay informed about the latest information on organic foods and have a political voice regarding our food, go to www.organicconsumers.org and sign up for the free e-newsletter. It's interesting, informative, and gives you opportunities to make your voice heard politically.

In addition to choosing organically grown food, check carefully to see if the vegetables and fruit have been irradiated. FDA requires that irradiated foods

Avoid the "Dirty Dozen"

The nonprofit research organization Environmental Working Group reports periodically on health risks posed by pesticides in produce. The group says you can cut your pesticide exposure by almost 90 percent by avoiding the top-twelve conventionally grown vegetables and fruit that are the most contaminated; purchase only organic for these twelve. Using this guide will help you make wise choices. Whenever you are on a cleansing program it is vitally important to consume food that is as pesticide free as possible. (You can also stay current on the "dirty dozen" by doing a websearch, since the list may change from time to time.)

THE DIRTY DOZEN (HIGHEST PESTICIDE LOAD)

• Peaches	100	• Potatoes	81
• Apples	96	• Cherries	75
• Celery	94	• Lettuce	69
• Sweet bell peppers	86	• Grapes (imported)	68
• Nectarines	84	• Pears	65
• Strawberries	83	• Spinach	60

THE CLEANEST TWELVE

• Avocado	1	• Sweet peas (frozen)	11
• Onions	1	• Kiwi fruit	14
• Sweet corn (frozen)	2	• Bananas	16
• Pineapple	7	• Cabbage	17
• Mango	9	• Broccoli	18
• Asparagus	11	• Eggplant	19

Note: Since carrots are used often in juice recipes, be aware that they are number thirteen, right after spinach at 57 pesticide load; therefore, it's important to buy organic carrots.

include labeling with either the statement "treated with radiation" or "treated by irradiation," along with the international symbol for irradiation, the Radura. Irradiation labeling requirements apply only to foods sold in stores. For example, irradiated spices or fresh strawberries should be labeled. But irradiation labeling is not required for restaurant foods. Irradiation, known as gamma-ray radiation, is used to kill pests and germs in stored food, which seems to improve the shelf life of the food, but it doesn't preserve your life. Even though the FDA allows its use, radiation doses for food decontamination can be up to five million times that of a typical chest X-ray. They may kill the bugs, but they also generate free radicals in the food, that when ingested, can damage your cells. In addition, the practice destroys vitamins and minerals.

Genetically Modified Foods

Whenever possible, avoid genetically modified foods, also known as GMs or GMOs. Scientists, doctors, and health educators in many sectors of the health industry have long warned about the possible deleterious effects of GM crops on the health of animals and humans. An Australian project to develop genetically modified peas with built-in pest resistance had to be abandoned after tests showed they caused allergic lung damage in mice. A similar situation occurred in the early 1990s when a strain of bioengineered soybeans was found to cause an allergic response in people with Brazil nut allergies.

A March 2007 article in the journal *Archives of Environmental Contamination and Toxicology* reported on a study that was commissioned by the environmental group Greenpeace in which rats were fed for ninety days on GM maize (corn) developed by the chemical giant Monsanto. The rats showed signs of toxicity in the liver and kidneys. In reporting on this study, *Scientific American* quoted a statement by Greenpeace spokesman, Arnaud Apoteker, saying, "It is the first time that independent research, published in a peer-reviewed journal, has proved that a GMO authorized for human consumption presents signs of toxicity."

A genetically modified organism (GMO) is an organism whose genetic material has been altered using bioengineering techniques. These GMO foods have raised concerns because they force genetic information across the protective species barrier in an unnatural way. In other words, nature does not sustain them. These new organisms are in many cases untested, yet they are on grocery store shelves everywhere without protective labeling. In other words, we may not know we are buying them.

The United States is the main supplier of GMO seeds

worldwide and the crops are virtually uncontrolled in this country. On the other hand, many countries around the world have banned their use, including many in the European Union that are fighting to keep their crops pure. Hungary, one of Europe's biggest grain producers, became the first country in Eastern Europe to ban GMO crops or foods when it outlawed the planting of maize seeds, marketed by Monsanto, in January 2005. As it stands now, we have about a 70 to 75 percent chance of picking a product with GMO ingredients without even realizing it. This is astounding! We need to take notice when we're selecting food to build our health, particularly if we are cleansing to remove toxins. We can each make our voice heard that we don't want GMO crops grown in the United States.

We can avoid GMO foods by becoming aware of which foods are most prone to genetic engineering and what products are made from them. To date, the biggest GM crops are soybeans and corn, from which thousands of processed foods are made. Look at the labels on all products you purchase to see if they contain corn flour or corn meal, soy flour, cornstarch, textured vegetable protein, corn syrup, or modified food starch. Check labels of soy sauce, tofu, soy beverages, soy protein isolate, soy milk, soy ice cream, margarine, soy lecithin, among dozens of other products. If it doesn't say organic for these foods, the chances are strong that it's GMO. It's particularly important to choose organic soy or corn products to ensure that they are not GMO. Aside from corn and soy, other GMO foods grown in the United States include cotton (cottonseed oil), canola, sugar beets, squash, and papaya. You can vote with your dollars by purchasing only products labeled organic, especially when it comes to foods and by-products of food that are likely to be grown from GMO crops.

Become an informed consumer. The FDA has refused to require labeling of genetically engineered foods, despite overwhelming American support for mandatory labeling. Since the agency has refused to protect consumers, some food companies are now taking action by labeling certain products or ingredients "non-GMO," which means "made without genetically modified organisms." The United States may soon be the only country in the world that does *not* require labeling of genetically engineered food.

Summary of Juicing for Life

Step 1. Continue eating whole foods, alkalizing foods, using organic, non-GMO, removing as many sources of toxicity as possible, drinking plenty of water, and eating at least 50 percent raw foods.

Step 2. Add fresh vegetable juices to your diet at least once or twice a day.

CHAPTER THREE

Fasting for Life

Fasting is an excellent way to lose weight and cleanse the body of toxins, but it is much more than that. Its virtues have been extolled for centuries by nearly every religious practice as a way to connect to something higher and more significant than one's self and the needs of one's body. Fasting can make you feel lighter, happier, healthier, and more focused. The air will seem clearer, colors brighter, and sights and sounds sharper and more beautiful.

Fasting literally means to abstain from all or certain types of food and drink. It can mean a lot of different things such as fasting from sugar, alcohol, coffee, meat, dairy, or whatever else one chooses to give up. There are many types of fasts and methods of fasting. Some of these methods are quite controversial. For instance, one type of fasting, known as total fasting, is to take nothing in by mouth — not food or water. I consider a total fast dangerous. Our bodies need two to two and a half quarts of water a day to function well. Without adequate water, dehydration can occur, electrolyte balance is disturbed, and the delicate tissues of the body can become damaged.

Another type is the water-only fast. This fast involves totally abstaining from all solid or liquid food and drinking only water. I don't recommend water-only fasting unless you've completed a number of cleansing programs and some vegetable-juice fasting beforehand, because fasting causes toxins to be rapidly released into the bloodstream. Without an ample supply of antioxidants from your diet, provided with vegetable juices, and/or supplements, the large amount of toxins released with fasting could damage your cells. Antioxidants bind to toxins and carry them out of the body so they don't cause damage. I use vegetable-juice fasting because vegetable juices are loaded with antioxidants and they are very alkalizing. This is a safe and effective way to cleanse the internal organs, tissues, and cells of your body. Vegetable-juice fasting supports detoxification by providing nutrients, with an abundance of antioxidants like vitamins C and E, beta-carotene, selenium, and various enzymes and phytochemicals that bind to and neutralize toxins.

When you fast, you are voluntarily setting aside the temptations of food, the ritual of eating, and the demands of your cravings. In exchange for the discipline of forgoing solid food for a period of time, you'll have a chance to reflect on the deeper aspects of your soul, such as your purpose, and what is truly important in life. Fasting can free you from addictions and dependencies of all kinds. It can give you the sense of control over your body that allows you to consider new ways of living and new possibilities. You'll see creative solutions to problems more clearly when you are not weighed down with the burden of food preparation and digestion. And your body and soul is given a chance to heal.

During Lent, the monks at some monasteries chant, "Through abstinence, what is tired and weak and sick becomes strong." This is actually true. You'll become stronger because of your fast. This might seem like an oxymoron, since we think of food as a key to strength. Indeed, healthy food does make you strong. But there is a place for abstinence from food as well in our rhythm of life, and fasting will also strengthen and renew your body and soul.

Fasting is energizing because you are resting your body from the work of digestion. Normally, about 30 percent of our overall energy expenditure is devoted to digestion.

Think of it — you'll have 30 percent more energy freed up just by not eating!   •

When you fast, this energy can be used for healing. Without solid food being ingested throughout the day, the body looks for new sources of fuel to burn for energy. It first draws on readily available glucose that is stored in the liver as glycogen. Next it turns to other sources like the fatty acids in fat cells and proteins that are most readily available. Then it turns to sick or damaged cells. The body is continually making new cells and breaking down old, sick, or damaged ones. Of the trillions of cells in our body, it is estimated that about one-fourth, or around three to eight hundred billion, are broken down and replaced daily. During fasting, the process of degrading sick cells is accelerated. Their raw materials are then recycled to be used either as energy or building blocks for new cells. Those that cannot be used are eliminated. This explains why skin starts to look so much younger and more vibrant during a fast and why the body starts getting well.

When you fast a few days, many cravings go away and thoughts about food usually diminish. You have time to focus on other things. This gives your body a chance to use its energy for clearing out old waste that has accumulated in both your body and mind. Many people report a spiritual experience during this time. Other people are simply joyful because they feel in control of their

appetite for the first time in years or are making prog-
ress on health improvement or weight management.

Just like many things that are good for us, fasting has
gotten a bad rap in our culture. We're so inundated with
advertising that tells us we have to constantly consume
food that the very idea of going without it — *on purpose* —
is contrary to everything we're conditioned to believe.

You may be thinking that fasting is something so
difficult that you can't possibly do it, or that it's only for
those super-disciplined people who don't suffer from
any of the challenges you've had when you tried fasting in the past. I understand, because I've been there.
However, I can promise you that fasting doesn't have to
involve unnecessary pain or discomfort. Let me encourage you to give it a try. Millions of people throughout
time have fasted successfully. And, thankfully, you don't
have to *white-knuckle* it through a difficult water fast. A
short vegetable-juice fast is something that almost anyone can do, including you. You can happily fast for a day
or two with fresh juices, smoothies, and cold soups and
feel good in the process. Later, if you choose, you can go
on a longer fast and enjoy even greater benefits.

Since fasting involves abstaining from food, many
people have a negative reaction when they think about it.
Some people focus on denial and the possibility of discomfort. Some are fearful of weakness or detox symptoms, but most of the symptoms are due to the release

of toxins that have accumulated through the years and something that will make our bodies sick in the long run. Release of toxins is exactly what we want our bodies to do. So don't worry. I'll show you how to prepare for a fast so detox symptoms should be minor and pass quickly. I'll help you through your fast with tips to make it easier and show you how to successfully break a fast. And the rewards you'll get will be great.

Michele's Story

I never wanted to try fasting because I believed it would make me feel weak and sick. Because I was diagnosed with hypoglycemia (low blood sugar), I believed that I had to eat something every few hours, especially protein. My only experience with fasting was when I would try to do some sort of cleansing routine for my colon or liver, which was usually very unpleasant because I did it incorrectly.

When I began to learn about all the wonderful benefits of fasting, I decided to try it. First I did a one-day juice fast that included fresh vegetable juices and some smoothies made with vegetable juice and avocados. I felt so good I decided to try it for another two days. After three days of vegetable-juice fasting I felt full of energy and very clear-headed. And I was grateful to be freed from the chore of having to think about what I had to prepare to eat and what not to eat each day. I lost several pounds, too, although this was not my reason for the fast. I was amazed at how good I felt and decided to try it again the next week. Although I had a few detox symptoms, like a headache and a little weakness periodically, most of the time I felt incredibly well and was able to do moderate exercises. After completing the fast, I increased the intensity and time of my workouts in the gym. I literally felt like running a marathon on some of the days. I also noticed greater mental clarity and spiritual focus.

For me it was important to lead up to my fast with proper preparation. Cherie recommended that I add daily vegetable juicing to my diet for about two weeks before the fast, plus I ate almost 80 percent of my food fresh and raw. I believe the preparation enabled me to get through the fast with minimal discomfort.

(Continued)

I've noticed that many of the symptoms that have plagued me for years are mostly gone, as long as I don't overeat. I no longer have digestive problems like constipation or acid reflux. My weight is normal and my energy is high. My skin is clear and bright and my mental clarity is great, even though I'm over fifty. I'm now a dedicated juice faster and I tell all my friends about it and encourage them to try it too.

Why Juice Fasting Helps Us Look Younger and Trimmer

Each of the trillions of cells in our body has a permeable membrane that enables it to take in nutrients and excrete waste. Cell membranes often become hardened, or rigid, thus the cells cannot properly excrete toxins that were previously trapped within them. Much of the reason for cell wall rigidity is because of the acidity of toxic waste that is caused by eating too much acid-producing food, constant stress, negative thoughts and emotions, and environmental toxins. The acidity in the fluids surrounding the cells changes them and they become hardened.

When the cells are not properly able to excrete the buildup of toxic and acidic waste, this condition affects their ability to produce energy. This is because the mitochondria, little structures within the cells that generate ATP (a form of chemical energy), become much less efficient at their assigned task of producing energy. The result is that we feel tired, worn-out, and lethargic and we start looking older.

Along comes vegetable-juice fasting to the rescue. It alkalizes the cells and the surrounding fluids so they can dump waste, while supplying antioxidant nutrients that help to neutralize the toxins. Fasting restores alkaline balance and enables cell walls to return to their ideal, permeable state. Once the cell membranes are softened, the process of dumping wastes is accelerated. Now the cells can again function at peak efficiency, something they may not have been able to do for many years.

Alkalizing and cleansing your body also helps you lose weight. The body is very intelligent. As we become more and more acidic, it sets up defense mechanisms to keep the damaging acid from entering our vital organs. We know that acid gets stored in fat cells. After all, if the acid comes into contact with our organs, it can damage tissues and cause cells to mutate. Also, the oxygen level drops in an acidic environment, which sets up an environment for cancer cells to thrive. And calcium becomes depleted in an acidic environment, which is a setup for osteoporosis. So as a defense mechanism, your body may actually make fat to protect you from an overly acidic internal environment. Those fat cells and cellulite deposits (that lumpy, bumpy orange-peel skin) may actually be packing up the acid to keep it at a safe distance from your organs. When your body starts dumping toxins, it can also let go of fat because it doesn't need it anymore. And, voila! That stubborn, hard-to-lose pudge just seems to melt away — sometimes quite rapidly. This fat loss may not be due as much to reduction in calories as it is to flushing away acidic waste. This truly is an "eat and grow thin" possibility.

The Physical Benefits of Fasting

- Increases energy and strength
- Detoxifies cells and tissues
- Assists in weight loss
- Improves mental clarity
- Restores alkaline balance
- Strengthens the immune system
- Helps prevent disease
- Tightens skin
- Smoothes wrinkles
- Lowers blood pressure
- Lowers cholesterol
- Lessens aches and pains
- Revitalizes organ systems
- Rests the gastrointestinal system
- Balances the nervous system
- Increases ease of movement
- Helps the lungs breathe more deeply

Preparing to Fast

If you decide to do a one-day juice fast then just jump right in and go for it! It doesn't have to be difficult, complicated, or take a lot of preparation. Almost anyone can do well on a one-day vegetable-juice fast and will feel better for it. If you've never fasted before, start with one day. Most people do best if they start out slowly and then add more fast days later on.

The following suggestions for fasting will help you tremendously if you decide to do two, three, or more days of fasting. There are people who routinely do five-to ten-day juice fasts, which is where many of the most transforming benefits are realized. Listen to your body if you decide to fast longer than three days. If you want to have a successful two- or three-day fast with all the benefits that have been described, it's best to prepare properly before you begin. I have found this to be a very important step for anyone who is beginning a fast. Should you decide to begin with a two- or three-day fast, it will help if you lead up to it. Follow the guidelines Making Wise Food Choices on page 35 in chapter one.

Additionally, one week before your fast, eat smaller portions. Most of us can get by on about half of our usual serving sizes, so it's a great idea to practice eating only enough to satisfy your hunger. Also, eat more raw vegetables and fruit, making about 75 to 80 percent of your diet raw. This will slowly help to detoxify and alkalize your body so you will have fewer detox symptoms when you fast.

Many people fail at fasting because they go straight into a water-only or juice fast without any preparation or transition. If you jump from the typical American diet into a several-day fast, you could feel quite sick and swear you'll never do that again. Lots of people do a "pig-out" before they start a fast; that's really not a good idea. Resist the temptation to have a big last supper before you fast. Ease into your fast and prepare for it.

Exercise is also important in any cleansing program.

If you are not accustomed to regular exercise, begin now by walking, bicycling, slow jogging, rebounding, or dancing. If you haven't had any exercise for a while, start with fifteen to thirty minutes and work up to more time. And ease into it with something not too strenuous like walking or rebounding. Competitive or intense workouts are not good starter exercises; you could end up so sore you wouldn't be able to exercise for quite a while. Also incorporate regular stretching exercises into your daily routine. And don't forget to take plenty of deep breaths throughout the day.

CONSIDER YOUR MOTIVES FOR FASTING

Do you just want to lose weight, or are you fasting for improved health and wellness, or for spiritual reasons? It helps to have a clear idea about your motives when you start. If you want to cleanse and purify your body so you can increase your energy, mental clarity, and spiritual growth, write it down to remind yourself later when you may have a weak moment.

Fasting requires discipline, commitment, and inner determination. If you're in the right frame of mind when you start, it will be much easier. There are always temptations to pull you away from your commitment. Your family and friends may offer you a tempting dish, telling you, "Just one bite won't hurt." That's why it helps to write down your reasons for fasting, or tell a friend who will support you or even join you. It also helps to get away for a while like to an institute or a spa that offers fasting (see Resources Guide). If this is not possible, then begin to clear your schedule. Say no to commitments for a few days. Turn off the radio, television, and computer. Remind yourself it's just for a little while. The world will actually go on functioning without you! If you have family or work commitments, try to minimize any extra involvement with the outside world.

Prepare yourself mentally and physically by meditating, reading, exercising, praying, or just being still. You might want to take a day of relaxation before you begin your fast so you can calm your body and mind and reflect on what you want to gain from your fast. You will be most successful if you seek peace and serenity while you fast.

WHO SHOULD NOT FAST

Fasting is safe and beneficial for most people, yet some people should not fast, and others should fast only with supervision.

- Diabetics, particularly those on insulin (choose option two on page 85)
- Anyone with hypoglycemia (although many with blood sugar imbalances do well on a short vegetable-juice fast, especially if it's modified — see option two on page 85)

- Children under eighteen (unless recommended by a health professional)
- People with anemia, wasting as with advanced stages of cancer, or extreme weakness
- Anyone with a very aggressive cancer; however, modified fasts may be appropriate (see option two on page 85).
- People with eating disorders like anorexia or bulimia
- Women who are pregnant or nursing
- Anyone with a serious health problem may need professional supervision
- Anyone with concerns about fasting should consult a health professional

How to Fast

Now that you have decided to fast for either one, two, three, or more days and you've set aside the time and cleared your schedule, you can relax and settle into the adventure of juice fasting. Make sure you have plenty of fresh organic vegetables and a few low-sugar fruits on hand such as lemon, lime, or green apples, so you don't have to go shopping on your fasting days.

You can drink as much vegetable juice as you like and as often as you like. Some people choose to make a variety of juices throughout the day; others prefer to make one big batch (several glasses) of juice at one time and sip on it throughout the day. It's up to you. If you do make the juice ahead of time, keep it in an airtight container to preserve as many of the enzymes and vitamins as possible.

TYPES OF JUICE FASTS

There are two basic versions of juice fasting: juice fasting with just juices; or a modified fast consisting of juices and blended cold soups and vegetable smoothies.

Option I: **Vegetable juices only.** Make any of the vegetable juice recipes in this book or your own combinations. The vegetable-juice fast gets the best results because adding avocado, as recommended for smoothies and cold soups in option two, can slow the detox process. However, choose option two if you have low blood sugar, diabetes, extreme fatigue, or any other condition where you need to have some protein each day, unless your doctor says you can't. Or you may want option two because you know that for emotional reasons, you would not fast otherwise.

Option 2: **Juices, cold soups, and vegetable smoothies.** A modified fast involves the use of fresh juices plus blender smoothies. This fast allows you to have more substantial and calorie-rich liquids, as long as they're blended or pureed. I often make vegetable juice and put it into the blender with an avocado to make a thicker mixture with a souplike consistency. The addition of the avocado will slow down the detoxification process, but it is still effective. Another option is to scoop out some of the pulp from the juicer, add a little juice, and eat it like a soup. Since the vegetables are already ground up, the pulp is much more easily digested.

What to Do During the Fast

Drink plenty of purified water. Be sure to get two to two and a half quarts of water in addition to the juice. The more water you consume, the easier it is for your body to flush away the waste. Drinking enough water takes some discipline, but stick with it. Drink more than enough to satisfy your thirst. Keep drinking and stay close to a bathroom.

Include herbal tea. Part of your water can be in the form of herbal tea and you can drink as much as you like. Beneficial herbal teas include dandelion root and nettles, which help cleanse the liver and kidneys. Milk thistle is extremely good for the liver. Peppermint is good for upset stomach and chamomile is relaxing. You can also purchase detox teas in health food stores or supermarkets in the nutrition center. If you buy herbal tea in bulk, steep one-half to one teaspoon in a pint of hot water for ten minutes, strain, and drink warm. Lemon may be added for flavor, but do not use any sweetener, except a small amount of stevia, if desired.

Avoid stimulants. Stay away from coffee, tobacco, alcohol, soda pop, sweets, and all other stimulants. A small amount of white or green tea can be tolerated well by most people, but it should be on the weak side.

Choose organic vegetables, herbs, and low-sugar fruit. Some of the best vegetables and fruit for cleansing are carrot, beet, lemon, lime, sprouts of all kinds, wheatgrass, celery, kale, green pepper, cucumber, parsley, asparagus, lettuce, spinach, collard greens, fennel, sweet potatoes, yams, garlic, ginger, grapefruit, and low-sugar apples like Granny Smith or pippin. Cabbage juice is also good, but it must be consumed immediately, as it does not store well.

Preparing Your Produce for Juicing

Wash everything well, even if it's organic. Organic produce is often still dirty and can have undesirable soil organisms or other contaminants on them. There are good vegetable washes available at health food stores and many grocery stores. You can also use sea salt in a sink full of water or food-grade hydrogen peroxide mixed in a basin of water.

Prepare the produce for juicing. Cut produce into pieces that will fit into your juicer's feed tube. Peel the produce when appropriate, such as grapefruit skin, which should not be consumed because of the volatile oils in the skin. Slowly feed the pieces into the feeding tube. For leafy greens like spinach, parsley, lettuce, or kale, bunch them up first, then push through slowly with something hard like a carrot. Parsley works best if rolled up in a lettuce or kale leaf. When finished juicing, you can strain the juice if desired, then pour into a glass and drink.

How to drink juice. You can chill it if you wish, but drinking it at room temperature is easier on the digestive system. Be sure to swish the juice around in your mouth to mix with saliva, which is necessary for digestion of the carbohydrates in the juice. Try not to gulp your juice down too quickly; sip it slowly.

What to Do During a Healing Crisis

Fasting can occasionally produce some negative symptoms because toxins are being moved out of storage places within the body and this release can cause some adverse symptoms. Detox symptoms are usually referred to as a healing crisis or the Herxheimer Reaction. This crisis is good, it just *feels* bad sometimes, but it will pass; it's actually a good sign that you're getting rid of a lot of harmful stuff. Some possible symptoms include headaches; bad breath; a coated or furry tongue; canker sores;

nausea, constipation, or diarrhea; skin eruptions; rashes; feelings of sadness, depression, or anger; backaches; muscle aches; light-headedness; weakness, or fatigue. You may experience one or more of these symptoms as you fast, but don't worry, they'll soon pass.

During a healing crisis, there are several things you can do to help yourself feel better:

- **Take a short nap or a rest break.** Sleep more than usual during a fast.
- **Drink extra water,** fresh vegetable juice, or herbal tea to flush out the toxins.
- **Exercise** by taking a short walk, stretching, bouncing on a rebounder, or using a lymphasizer, all of which help the lymphatic system remove toxins more rapidly.
- **Take plenty of deep breaths.**
- **Take an enema** or get a colonic (see page 155).
- **Use fiber,** if constipated. Psyllium husks or flax fiber act as a bulk laxative and can help move toxins through the colon more efficiently. Add one or two teaspoons of fiber to either juice or water, stir thoroughly, and drink immediately before it gets too thick. Use this three times a day during the first few days of a fast. Senna tea is also helpful. (See other suggestions in chapter five, Colon Cleansing for Vibrant Health).
- **Dry skin brushing** is also good at this time, as it

allows toxins to escape through the skin, which is the largest organ of elimination. Get a natural bristle bath brush and brush the skin in an upward motion.

- **Take a dry or infrared sauna** to sweat out more toxins. (Sweating is the only way to get rid of plastic toxins.)
- **Take care of your body and soul.** Rest, read a good book, call a fasting partner, meditate, or pray.
- **Positive self-talk.** Congratulate yourself for doing something great for your body. Tell yourself that you are getting healthier and more vibrant because of your efforts at fasting. If you don't feel as well as you'd like, tell yourself this too shall pass. Remind yourself that on the other side is great healing, vibrant health, a trimmer body, and a renewed soul.
- **Remember that fasting is a choice** that you made to help your body come up to a higher level of health. No one is making you do this; you chose it for yourself.

Breaking the Fast

This part is as important as the fast itself, and more important in some ways, in that if you break it with a big steak or a pizza, you could do your body more harm than good and undo all the good you just did. And you could end up with a terrible stomachache. I know. Once, I broke my three-day juice fast with a restaurant salad bar and a few bites of seafood. But that was too much and I was doubled over in pain. Eat vegetables, nuts and seeds, a little low-sugar fruit, and some vegetable soups for a day or two after your fast and make sure to eat plenty of those foods raw. Chew everything well. Let your digestive system gradually return to normal. After the fast, the toxins that have been released may still be finding their way out through the channels of elimination, especially the colon, so it's best not to add too much food back into your diet right away, and certainly not heavy animal proteins that are hard to digest. Just as you resisted the temptation to have a "last big supper," resist having a large meal soon after a fast.

Introduce heavy foods like proteins back into your diet very slowly in small portions. You will probably find that you want less food, so now is not the time to go out with your friends to an all-you-can-eat buffet. If you go out for social or business reasons right after breaking your fast, you can ask for a special salad that has only vegetables, or get a vegetable soup, or a vegetarian meal. Avoid the bread and butter. Order sparkling water or herbal tea with lemon or lime to drink.

How Do I Detox When I'm Busy and Other Frequently Asked Questions

Many people have asked me numerous questions through the years about how to make detox programs work for them. Here are some of the most often asked questions and answers.

(Continued)

How do I fit detox programs into a busy schedule? The best way to begin a detox program is on the weekend when you have a little more time to organize what you need. Prepare ahead for the workweek at this time. Most of the programs are just seven days and you can get through nearly anything for a week. But you do need to be ready for the busy days by shopping in advance and preparing as much of the food as possible in advance. Remember, it's only seven days, but seven important days that could have a great impact on your health.

Will I have low energy and not be able to do anything? Most people find that their energy is not low and they are able to do what they need to each day. But if your energy does become low, then take it easy. If you had a cold or flu, you'd probably have to slow down. The detox programs are very important for your health, and will help you prevent colds and flus. If you have to take it a little slower for a few days, you're doing your body a big favor in the long run and it will reward you with greater energy in the future.

Will the programs taste bad? Most of the detox programs incorporate fresh juice, which tastes great. And many of the other recipes also taste good. A few herbal tinctures can have a strong taste. But nearly everyone is able to complete all the programs without a problem.

How do I know if these programs are for me? The detox programs are for everyone. We all need them because we're all bombarded with toxins in our air, soil, food, and water that interfere with our biochemical processes and contribute to weight gain, low energy, aging, sickness, and disease. Detoxing the body produces both immediate and long-term benefits.

How do I tailor the programs to fit my schedule and needs? First, try to pick a week when you don't have too many obligations or move things around to free up more time. Prepare foods in advance to take to work. Let your family and friends know this is your week to take care of yourself and you won't be joining them for certain events or meals. If some parts of the program just seem impossible, do your best.

What happens if I get off track? As you detox your body, the important work of detoxification builds, day after day. If you cheat even one time in the middle, you'll either greatly slow the detox or stop it. You don't want to do that when you've worked hard to get to that place. However, if you do get off track, don't stop completely; keep going. You may want to add an extra day or two, depending on how off track you got.

How can I feed a family and stay on the program? It may take some willpower if you have to make meals for your family and special food for you. But you can do it. It's only for a week for most of the programs. If there's someone else in your family who can prepare meals during this time, it will help you a lot if they'd agree to make all the meals for the time you're on your detox program. Otherwise, prepare your food and theirs and eat your food while they eat theirs, may be in different places. Or find what works for you.

What if I have to do business over a meal during the detox? You can order a big vegetable main course salad without any animal products in it. Nearly every restaurant in America will prepare this kind of salad. You can ask for oil and vinegar for the dressing. You can order hot water and lemon or sparkling water and lemon or lime. This makes a great meal and it may impress the people you are eating with. After all, you're eating really healthy and most people wish they had that kind of willpower. If you're in the middle of a juice fast, you'll need to pass on the salad. Just explain what you're doing.

What do I do at parties and during holidays? You can drink sparkling water and lemon or just plain water, if need be. Most parties have a vegetable tray, so you can munch on the veggies. But make sure you eat what you need to before the party so you won't be hungry and tempted. Regarding holidays, it's best to avoid a detox program during major holidays. It's just too difficult for most people. But if you're battling a life-threatening illness, then you may want to embark on a detox program at this time so you won't be tempted to eat the wrong foods. For holidays that aren't major, this might be a time to do a detox program since you should have an extra day or two off from work where you can focus on your cleanse program and taking care of yourself.

Which detox program should I start with? I recommend you begin with the Colon Cleanse, then move to the Liver/Gallbladder Cleanse, and finally the Kidney Cleanse. If you need any of the specialized cleanses, you can follow with those that apply to you. At any time, you can benefit from a one- to three-day vegetable-juice fast.

A Sample One-Day Juice Fast Guide

Below is a sample menu for a day of juice fasting. This menu can be modified or amended to suit your individual needs and tastes. You can follow this program for one, two, three days, or more. If you're doing the modified juice fast, you can take any of these juices, put them in your blender, and add an avocado. This will make a great cold soup that is delicious and sustaining.

BREAKFAST

THE BREAKFAST ZINGER

3 to 4 medium carrots
1 small beet with leaves
1/2 cucumber
1/2 small or medium lemon
  (peeled if not organic)

1/2- to 1-inch piece fresh
  gingerroot
1/2 green apple (optional)

Juice the carrots, beet, cucumber, lemon, and ginger. If you decide to use apple, remember that it will add extra fruit sugar (avoid if diabetic or hypoglycemic). Cut the apple into pieces and feed into the juicer tube after the ginger. Stir the juice, and pour into a glass. Serve at room temperature or chilled.

MIDMORNING BREAK

THE WALDORF

*3 to 4 leaves of romaine
   lettuce
3 stalks organic celery
   with leaves
1/2 cucumber*

*1/4 small or medium
   lemon (peeled if not
   organic)
1/2 green apple (optional)*

Bunch up the lettuce one leaf at a time; push through with celery, cucumber, and lemon. If you decide to use apple, remember that it will add extra fruit sugar (avoid if diabetic or hypoglycemic). Cut the apple into pieces and feed into the juicer tube. Stir the juice, and pour into a glass. Serve at room temperature or chilled.

LUNCH

SPINACH TOWER OF POWER

*1 to 2 cups organic
   spinach
1 handful parsley
3 to 4 medium carrots*

*1 stalk organic celery with
   leaves
1/2 beet with stems and
   leaves*

Bunch up the spinach and parsley, and push them through the feed tube with the carrots, celery, and beet. Stir the juice, and pour into a glass. Serve at room temperature or chilled.

HAPPY HOUR

SOUTHWESTERN COCKTAIL

*1 medium vine-ripened
    tomato
1/2 medium organic
    cucumber
1/4 cup cilantro (use
    parsley if cilantro is too
    strong tasting for you)*

*1/4 small or medium lime
    or lemon, peeled if not
    organic
Dash of hot sauce
    (optional)*

Cut the tomato into sections that fit your juicer's feed tube. Cut the cucumber in half lengthwise. Bunch up the cilantro, and push through the feed tube with the tomato, cucumber, and lime or lemon. Pour the juice into a glass, add the hot sauce (as desired), and stir. Serve at room temperature or chilled.

DINNER

Option 1:

Any of the juice recipes from chapter ten.

Option 2:

CHERIE'S AWESOME ENERGY SOUP

*4 to 5 medium carrots
1 cucumber
2 stalks celery
1/2 lemon, peeled*

*1- to 2-inch piece of ginger-
    root, peeled if not
    organic
1 avocado, peeled and
    seed removed*

Juice the carrots, cucumber, celery, lemon, and ginger. Add the juice to a blender and then add the avocado. Blend until smooth. Pour the mixture into a bowl and eat with a spoon. Delicious and nourishing, this is a great recipe for those with hypoglycemia or diabetes.

BEDTIME SNACK

SWEET DREAMS TONIGHT

2 romaine lettuce leaves
1 handful parsley
4 carrots

3 organic celery stalks
   with leaves

Bunch up the lettuce leaves and parsley, and push through the feed tube with the carrots and celery. Stir the juice, and pour into a glass. Serve at room temperature or chilled, as desired.

Juice Fasting Recap

Incorporate the vibrant health recommendations in chapter one for one to two weeks before the fast and follow the fasting guidelines.

Step 1: Eat whole, alkalizing, organic foods and eat 50 to 75 percent raw foods. Two days before fasting, increase to 75 to 80 percent raw.

Step 2: Remove as many sources of toxicity as possible.

Step 3: Drink plenty of purified water—2 to 2 1/2 quarts per day.

Step 4: Add fresh vegetable juices to your diet at least once or twice a day.

Step 5: Embark on a one- to three-day vegetable-juice fast.

Step 6: Break your fast wisely.

CHAPTER FOUR

Detoxing for Life

Thinking about our organs of elimination can be about as appealing as discussing how the clothes dryer's lint trap works or why the garbage disposal makes certain noises. But we all know these appliances are hot topics when they stop working efficiently or completely break down. The same is true for our organs of elimination. The trouble is, oftentimes we don't know they aren't working well; we just know we don't feel well.

A sound program of periodic detoxification will engage all the major organs in your body's detoxification system—intestines, liver, kidneys, skin, gallbladder, lungs, and lymphatics, to improve your health and prevent disease. You could consider detoxification as being like a thorough spring housecleaning that is taking place on the inside. Just as you need to deep clean your home occasionally and really dig into corners, drawers, and closets where dirt and unwanted items accumulate, so you need to dig deeper when it comes to the organs of elimination and cleanse them thoroughly to eliminate the waste and toxins that have accumulated over time.

You could think of internal housecleaning in a creative new way: You have a good internal built-in vacuum system (the intestinal tract), a washing machine (the liver), lots of cleaning rags and fluids (the lymph and blood), a drain (the kidneys), a fan to blow out stale air and toxins (the lungs), and plenty of natural cleaning products (fresh juices loaded with antioxidants and other supplemental nutrients) that will help you get the job done right.

The body is designed to detoxify a host of waste products. All you have to do is assist with the process by keeping out as many sources of toxins as possible while providing the right materials to assist in detoxification by providing good nutrition and nutrient supplementation. And you can work on each of the major organs of elimination separately and in the right order — first the colon, then the liver and gallbladder, and finally the kidneys. Detoxing these primary organs of elimination will enable the supporting channels — the lungs, lymph, and blood — to function at their maximum capacity.

It's estimated that on average people have at least five to ten pounds of accumulated toxic waste in their cells, tissues, and organs. (That's five to ten pounds we could really feel great about dropping!) Toxic substances that accumulate throughout the body can weaken and congest our organs and systems of elimination. As we've already seen, these substances come from a number of sources such as the environment, unhealthy food choices, and internal by-products of metabolism, called endotoxins. Toxic substances such as chemicals, pesticides, drug residues, heavy metals, food additives, along with by-products from food digestion, as well as yeasts, fungus, and parasites can pile up in our system like logs jamming a river. If they are not broken down and eliminated, they are stored in the intestines, gallbladder, kidneys, liver, skin, bone, and fat cells, making us sick, weak, overweight, and unable to fight off infections. And toxic molecules, known as free radicals, damage our cells, accelerating aging and creating many health problems. This is why it's so crucial to periodically cleanse your body.

With over eighty-seven thousand new chemicals produced every year, we are exposed to thousands of toxins on a daily basis! Where do they go? More important, how do we get rid of them? The next two sections will give you a quick outline to help you understand how the body stores them, what happens with toxic buildup, and what your body does to detoxify and eliminate these toxins.

Fighting the Free Radical Battle

Free radicals are toxic molecules that bombard our healthy cells and cause damage. They are unstable molecules that have lost an electron, so they are quick to react with other compounds, trying to gain stability by capturing an electron from somewhere else. This sets off a chain reaction as the next molecule loses its electron and becomes a free radical itself. The process then begins to cascade, eventually resulting in the disruption of living cells.

The production of free radicals can be likened to the rusting of metal, which occurs when the metal reacts with oxygen in the air. This process is called "oxidation." The same thing happens inside us, as our body's molecules are also vulnerable to oxidation. This internal oxidation is what produces the free radicals that contribute to numerous health conditions such as lack of energy and stamina, a less than optimal immune system, damaged cells, and premature aging.

Some free radicals are a normal result of biochemical processes and can easily be handled by our body's many defenses. However, nutritional and environmental factors such as pollution, radiation, pesticides, trans fats, and polyunsaturated fats in our diet can cause excessive free radical activity that can cause damage.

Detoxification helps fight this free radical battle in two important ways: first, by removing the source of excess toxicity and free radicals; and second, by contributing an abundant and powerful supply of antioxidants that attack the free radicals and neutralize them.

Where Have All the Toxins Gone?

Toxins are a bit like criminals; they hole up anywhere they can find a place to hide. They hang out in cells, tissues, and organs. They can be found especially in fat cells, and in the liver, kidneys, and large and small intestines. They hide in the mucus lining of the lungs and sinuses. And they are distributed into the cells and tissues of the brain where they can cause a lot of cognitive and emotional problems. When the organs and systems of elimination get behind in their work, there's a backup into the supporting systems just like dirty water backs up in a stopped-up sink. First the intestines build up mucus and putrefaction and nutrients are not properly absorbed; then poisons are absorbed back into the bloodstream. The liver becomes overwhelmed and congested and our blood is not cleansed properly so more toxins get into the bloodstream. The filtration system in the kidneys works hard to excrete toxic-laden urine, but they become overwhelmed, too, and some waste is recirculated.

This downward spiral affects more than just the elimination system. Toxins are shunted off to storage in fat cells so our organs will be protected from the acidity, since toxins are almost always acidic, and the body holds on to fat as a protection. Consequently, we have difficulty losing weight. These acidic pollutants collect in cells, tissues, and the fluids between the cells, making cellular metabolism inefficient at best. They can also show up as cellulite. And they can clog our skin, lungs, and the passages of the lymphatic system. The result of this toxic overload is sickness, tiredness, bad skin, and eventually disease.

Flush Away the Cellulite

It's not just another fat. Simply put, cellulite is irregular fat deposits. Essentially, this fat is trapped within connective tissues and the affected areas are full of fluid, toxins, lymph, and waste. These dimples and bumps are usually found on the thighs, hips, and buttocks, and most of us aren't very happy about them. Infuriatingly, many dieters find that no matter how hard they work at weight loss, exercise, and strict diet, this stuff sticks to the thighs like caramel on an apple—even when they've dropped down a size or two.

Because it's quite different from your garden-variety kind of pudge, cellulite has to be tackled in a unique way. Cellulite is associated with poorly functioning blood vessels, constipation, poor lymphatic drainage, and toxicity. If blood vessels are weak and sluggish, toxins will accumulate quickly, making it difficult for the body to burn fat in the affected areas. Constipation contributes to cellulite because it causes wastes and toxins to remain in the body rather than being eliminated. A sluggish, poor-functioning colon means that toxic wastes are not eliminated, and this affects the efficiency of organs such as the liver and kidneys.

Consuming sugar, refined salt (sodium chloride), caffeine, alcohol, tobacco, unhealthy fats and oils, and refined carbohydrates is taxing on your systems of elimination. This makes it much harder for your body to eliminate waste—and far easier for fat to get stored as cellulite. Some experts believe it's toxins that cause this fat to become trapped and held in one spot in the first place.

This kind of fat can't be eradicated just by eating healthy foods or by exercise. Though creams, lotions, or lymphatic drainage massage may help a little, they will not wipe away the lumps. You can rub, massage, and wrap this fat in seaweed every day of your life, but this stuff is not going to disappear unless you cleanse your body, especially your colon and liver, and improve your circulation and metabolism, get your lymph moving, and nourish your body from within. (One particular exercise machine known as a lymphasizer [swing machine] is particularly helpful [see Resources Guide]). Also, as you boost your metabolism, your circulatory and lymphatic systems will work better, and you'll increase your chances of shifting the bulges.

Changing your diet and detoxifying your body is key to eradicating cellulite. I know firsthand. You've got to flush out the toxins—plain and simple. It's also important to nourish and condition the areas affected in order to strengthen blood vessels and tissues and step up circulation. When toxins are removed and blood vessels and surrounding tissues are nourished, then it is possible for the fat to be used as energy. Your thighs don't have to look like a pitted golf ball any longer, and you can be trimmer *and sleeker* with the help of the cleansing programs.

What Causes Toxic Buildup?

Environmental toxins from the air, soil, and water bombard us — substances such as pesticides, herbicides, industrial chemicals and solvents, ionizing radiation, and other chemicals. Free radicals assault us further and weaken our ability to fight off viruses, bacteria, parasites, and cancer cells.

In addition, most of us eat too much sugar, refined carbohydrates, such as white flour products, fast food, junk food, fried food, and too much food period, which overwhelms our body's capacity to keep up with the work of digestion, assimilation, and detoxification of all that stuff. Then we drink too much alcohol, take medications, and ingest too many chemicals like preservatives, pesticides, and additives in commercial foods. Couple that with emotional toxicity such as fear, stress, worry, and anxiety and we have a full-blown toxic overload.

Looking deeper at some of these toxic sources, we see things we don't tend to think about as being toxic such as prescription and over-the-counter drugs. Pharmaceutical companies spend billions of dollars marketing drugs that frequently lead to side effects that are worse than the conditions they were meant to treat. These prescription and over-the-counter medications further contribute to a big toxic load on our liver that affects the entire body. The Centers for Disease Control and Prevention

(CDC) reports that poisoning from prescription drugs has become the second-largest cause of unintentional deaths in the United States. In *Morbidity and Mortality Weekly Report*, researchers stated that deaths from prescription drugs rose from 4.4 per 100,000 people in 1999 to 7.1 per 100,000 in 2004.

It's important to avoid prescription and over-the-counter drugs as much as possible. When a doctor prescribes a medication, it's a good idea to get a second opinion, preferably from a doctor who specializes in natural medicine such as a naturopath. Always look for a natural alternative remedy you can try first and lifestyle changes you can make to correct your health issues. This could make a huge difference in your health — both immediate and long-term.

Recently, I worked with a woman who had very high cholesterol. Her doctor wanted to prescribe cholesterol-lowering drugs, which she didn't feel comfortable taking. She opted for dietary changes and a red yeast rice supplement (rice that has been fermented by red yeast) under the supervision of a medical doctor. Within a short period of time her cholesterol went down to a healthy range and she was able to completely avoid drugs.

It's also important to avoid preservatives in our food. The Federal Food and Drug Administration (FDA) has now approved the spraying of viruses on all cold cuts to kill bacteria. Additionally, it has allowed cancer warnings to be pulled off of saccharine because it has been found to cause cancer only in high amounts. The FDA has allowed refined food manufacturers to put "No Trans Fats" on the food labels if there is less than 0.5g/serving and so manufacturers have changed serving sizes to avoid consequences. In small amounts, little bits of each of these additives may not sound like much, but added with all the other poisons we are exposed to on a daily basis, they do add up and place an incredible burden on our body's capacity to detoxify everything. Plus, no one has any idea about their interaction and what toxic by-products are created as a result.

The goal is to read labels and avoid everything with preservatives in it, as much as you possibly can. If you don't know what those strange-sounding words mean, don't buy it. When the label says less than 0.5g/serving of trans fats, avoid it. This will mean that you avoid a lot of packaged and processed food and opt for much more fresh food.

Sources of Toxicity

- Prescription drugs
- Additives from refined foods
- Aluminum and mercury from vaccines
- Mercury from amalgam fillings
- Biotoxins from mold or fungus
- Environmental toxins from paint, carpets, new furniture
- Home cleaning products like oven cleaners and toilet bowl cleaners
- Polishes for furniture and floors
- Air fresheners (sprays/solids)
- Antibacterial cleaners and soaps
- Dry-cleaning products
- Carpet and upholstery cleaners

Do You Have Signs of Toxicity?

When the major organs of elimination—intestinal tract, liver, and kidneys—are not working properly, your blood gets congested with chemical toxins, poisons, and other undesirable waste products. If these organs are clean and working efficiently, toxins will be filtered out and removed. When they remain in the body, they cause symptoms of toxic overload. These symptoms are many and varied, and they affect people in different ways, depending on genetic makeup, weaknesses in certain organs, strength of the immune system, and emotional and mental states. For example, impure blood circulating through the brain can cause mental and emotional distress, depression, anxiety, and neurological diseases.

Common Symptoms of Toxic Overload

- Lack of energy and fatigue
- Weakness
- Aches and pains
- Headaches
- Weight gain
- Inability to lose weight
- Irritability
- Emotional and mental problems
- Constipation
- Acid reflux
- Bloating and gas
- Indigestion
- Sinus problems
- Cellulite
- Trouble sleeping
- Restlessness
- Stressful feelings
- Dizziness
- Visual problems
- Skin problems
- Arthritis
- Hormone imbalances
- Premature aging

From the list above you can see that toxic overload contributes to a host of ailments in our modern lives. For instance, constipation and acid reflux are problems that can be attributed to poor diet and toxicity, which affects many people. These conditions have become so prevalent that over-the-counter laxatives and antacids are among the most marketed drugs in this country. Chronic Fatigue Syndrome (CFS) is another example of a condition that some doctors now believe is related to body toxicity. Many alternative medical doctors have found that cleansing the body of toxins is necessary to reverse CFS. (I'll attest to that firsthand; read my story in the introduction.) Toxicity is also at the root of many other ailments we're suffering from in the United States, such as cancer, allergies, autoimmune diseases, yeast infections, stomach problems, multiple chemical sensitivities, and other environmental illnesses.

Detoxification: Your Path to Vibrant Health

Your body has amazing processes for removing toxic substances or transforming them into harmless by-products. It's something our bodies do as part of their normal functioning. Because the body is its own healer, detoxification is part of its normal function, like breathing or digestion. It clears out toxins by eliminating them through the colon, liver, kidneys, lungs, skin, lymph, and blood.

The idea of assisting the body in detoxification is not a modern invention. Cultures throughout history have practiced cleansing through fasting, the use of herbs, enemas, and various colon-cleansing programs. But only in the past few decades has detoxification become crucial for everyone who lives in a modern culture. There are just too many sources of contamination, toxicity, and chemical buildup to ignore their effects. In his book *The Detox Miracle Sourcebook,* Dr. Robert Morse says detoxification is "a system for removing the causes of disease, not a system of treatment or a way to remove symptoms. It involves the understanding that the body is the healer."

The detox programs in the next chapters will help you remove the causes of disease, and if you are ill, detoxing can help you restore your body to the balance it was meant to have. Your energy and vitality will be renewed, you'll lose fat and cellulite, stubborn symptoms will lessen or disappear, and you'll achieve the glow of health and vitality that may have been eluding you for a long time. The good news is that we have built-in processes for dealing with toxins, poisons, chemicals, yeasts, parasites, and internal by-products of metabolism. We just need to do our part by supporting our organs of elimination through cleansing.

Benefits of Detoxifying

- Weight loss
- Cellulite reduction
- Increased energy
- Fewer wrinkles and age spots
- Improved immune function
- Blood purification
- Neutralization and elimination of free radicals and other toxins
- Optimal digestive function
- Reduced cravings (e.g., sugar, salt, junk foods, alcohol, and nicotine)

The Organs of Elimination

There are five primary organs of elimination: the intestines, liver, kidneys, lungs, and skin. Additionally, there are three supporting channels: the gallbladder, lymphatic system, and blood. The colon, liver, and kidneys are the primary organs of elimination in the digestive system. These organs are responsible for expelling toxins, either by excreting them directly or neutralizing them so they are no longer toxic. The main way they are excreted is through the colon as feces and through the kidneys as urine. Meanwhile, the supporting channels, gallbladder, lymphatic system, and blood, help to move the toxins and their by-products out of the body through bile, lymph, and blood.

The process breaks down when the intestinal tract becomes so clogged and congested that it is unable to properly eliminate waste. As you start the cleansing process, it's a good idea to first unclog these "pipes" with the colon cleanse. Next, cleanse and support the liver because it is the main organ of detoxification, and is responsible for deactivating and removing toxic chemicals from the body. If it is compromised and weak, then it's unable to fulfill its proper role in detoxification and toxins are stored away in places like that bumpy pudge on our thighs until the liver can get caught up again. Then cleanse the kidneys. And when you've completed your cleanses, you'll feel and look like a new person.

THE FUNCTIONS OF THE DIGESTIVE SYSTEM

There are two main functions of the digestive system. The first part is digestion and absorption of food. The second part is elimination of waste. Here's an overview of the organs that might help you understand what's going on.

The Intestinal Tract: Your Internal Plumbing

There are two main components of the intestinal tract — the small intestine and the large intestine, or colon. The intestines are coiled up inside the belly and stretch out to about twenty-six feet. That's a lot of surface area to allow absorption of nutrients and water to take place. Over 90 percent of all the nutrients we consume are absorbed in the small intestine, which makes it a key digestive organ.

The Small Intestine. The small intestine is made up of three segments: duodenum, jejunum, and ileum. The first section, the duodenum, is only about a foot or so long. This is where most of the minerals are absorbed from food. The next section is called the jejunum. It's longer — about eight feet. Here is where carbohydrates, protein, and water-soluble vitamins are absorbed. The final twelve-foot section is known as the ileum and is responsible for the absorption of fat, bile salts, cholesterol, and fat-soluble vitamins. Since the small intestine is responsible for extracting most of the nutrients from food, it's vitally important that it stays healthy and clean. Imbalances and congestion will interfere with its ability to sustain the body's nutritional needs. Many times people can eat reasonably well, yet they are not well nourished because of an improperly functioning small intestine.

The Large Intestine. The last five-foot portion of the intestine is known as the large intestine, or the colon. Food passes down this part of the digestive tract on its way to the anus, where it's excreted as feces. Along the way, it goes through three segments: the ascending colon, which connects to the end of the small intestine; then the transverse colon, which travels across the belly on top of the coiled-up small intestine; and finally, it heads down the left side of our body in what is called the descending colon. At the very end, the descending colon attaches to the rectum, which holds the feces before sending it out through the anus.

When food comes out of the small intestine it passes through a one-way valve called the ileocecal valve. At this point the food is called "chyme," and can be described as a thick mass of partially digested food and gastric secretions. It now enters the ascending colon, which is on the right side of the body. It's called "ascending" because it connects to the small intestine at a point toward the lower part of our abdomen, then moves up to the top of the coiled mass of the small intestine that is in the lower abdomen, transverses across the top, right to left, then descends down the left side. (This information may be helpful as you embark on the colon-cleansing program in the next chapter.)

As the chyme moves on, it heads across the transverse colon, where liquid and some final nutrients are extracted. It's here that the stool is formed into a semisolid state. More water is extracted as it travels along, gradually getting firmer as it moves toward the descending colon. The stool itself is typically about two-thirds water, insoluble fiber, and food products, and one-third living and dead bacteria. This mixture then enters the lowest portion of the bowel, which is called the sigmoid colon, and empties into the rectum for excretion.

The Colon: Our Waste-Disposal System. The colon, also known as the bowel, is a crucial organ of elimination — it is our body's waste-disposal system. If it is not working properly, our health suffers. The primary job of the bowel is to get rid of waste and toxic materials. It moves this material through the intestinal tract by a process known as peristalsis, which is a kind of rhythmic wave of contraction. If all is going well, the food from the small intestine enters the colon within about eight to ten hours after being consumed. The colon is filled with billions of microorganisms like friendly bacteria, yeast, and fungus; and although they live throughout the digestive system, most of them reside in the colon. A normal colon can have as much as four pounds of these microorganisms. One type is known as "friendly bacteria," because they are friends of our body and necessary for the proper breakdown of proteins, as well as the synthesis of certain vitamins.

In addition to the friendly guys, the colon also has "neutral" and "unfriendly" bacteria. In a healthy person, there is a ratio of roughly 80 percent friendly and neutral bacteria to 20 percent unfriendly bacteria. The balance of good and bad bacteria can be disrupted by various factors, but particularly by the overuse of antibiotics. When the bacteria are out of balance and bad bacteria outnumber the good, the unfriendly opportunists begin to take over, producing too many endotoxins that can be as toxic as most of the external toxins (exotoxins) from the environment.

These "bad" guys act on the undigested food in our gut producing toxic chemicals and gases that can damage the mucus lining of the intestines, leading to intestinal toxemia. These potent chemicals include acetaldehyde, formaldehyde, alcohol, ammonia, skatoles, indoles, hydrogen sulfide, methane gas, carbon dioxide, and free radicals. Once the intestinal lining is damaged, it becomes more permeable, often causing a condition known as leaky gut syndrome. The unhealthy waste products can now leak out of the gut and get reabsorbed into the bloodstream, where they affect both our physical and mental health. Because these substances are extremely toxic, a bowel movement every eight to twelve hours — or two or three times a day — is ideal for good health. Most people in our society have far less than the ideal, which is a bowel movement after each meal.

Good bowel health is dependent on sufficient fiber and water in the diet so the stool can move freely through the intestines. The longer the stool remains in the intestinal tract, the harder it becomes, because water will continually be absorbed. A dehydrated stool becomes hard and compacted and is thus difficult to eliminate. Eating a poor diet that is low in fiber and water causes the feces to remain in the gut longer and longer. Also, being deficient in magnesium and vitamin C can contribute to constipation. The longer transit time, the greater the chance that the bad bacteria will overtake the friendly ones and the gut will become foul smelling and toxic. A strong-smelling stool or intestinal gas indicates increased fermentation and putrefaction.

The intestinal tract tries to protect itself from the constant exposure to toxic substances like drugs, environmental chemicals, food additives, refined carbohydrates (white flour acts like glue in the intestines), and heavy metals by creating mucus on the intestinal wall. As mucus builds up on the lining, toxins, yeasts, and parasites stick to it, until it becomes something called "putrefactive debris." This prevents the proper assimilation of nutrients and contributes to toxins entering the bloodstream.

In summary, the intestines feed our cells, tissues, and organs. If they are congested and contaminated, it will affect the health of our blood and lymph, causing them to be filled with impurities that are carried throughout the body. This is why a periodic program of cleansing for the bowel is so important to prevent waste from backing up into our entire system.

The Liver: Our Waste-Processing Plant

Since the liver is the body's main organ of the detoxification, we need it to be well functioning to survive this toxic planet. It works day and night filtering toxins, chemicals, and poisons from the blood, detoxifying anything that is dangerous to our system, then neutralizing and eliminating the substances. It is the largest organ inside our body, weighing between three and five pounds, making it even bigger than the brain. It's responsible for more jobs than any other organ — about five hundred in all. It's the busiest and hardest working organ we have. If you put your hand on the right side of your abdomen, just under the diaphragm, you can feel it just slightly under the ribs. Think of it carrying out all these hundreds of vital functions and be thankful that it's working to keep you well and strong.

Every minute about two quarts of blood are delivered to the liver via the hepatic artery and the portal vein — that's about one hundred gallons of blood every day. This is an amazing figure, considering that our bodies have a total of about five quarts of blood in all. Oxygenated blood comes in from the hepatic artery, and deoxygenated blood comes from the portal vein carrying nutrients that have been absorbed. The liver extracts life-giving nutrients and oxygen from the blood, as well as toxic chemicals and waste products. The nutrients are processed for energy, and the toxins are prepared for elimination. Richard Anderson, ND, author of *The Liver: Cleansing and Rejuvenating the Vital Organ*, says, "We cannot be healthy or recover from illness without a strong, clean, well-functioning liver. The life, health, and vitality of every single organ, gland, and cell are absolutely dependent upon the liver."

The liver gets overwhelmed when it can't get rid of a lot of waste quickly enough. These toxic substances and waste products lodge in the cells and tissues, or they get shunted off for storage in fat cells. Colds, flu, rashes, skin eruptions, headaches, bladder infections, or other symptoms may develop as the body tries to maintain homeostasis by attempting to clean things out through the skin, lungs, and kidneys. If we take drugs to suppress these symptoms, or cure our cold or flu, the toxins remain, but are driven deeper into the tissues. Therefore, when we're sick, it's always best to treat our bodies with natural products and support our liver and immune system.

The Liver's Important Jobs

Of all the important jobs that the liver performs every day, the following are the most important for maintaining health:

- Regulates protein metabolism—necessary for hormones, enzymes, and structural components
- Regulates carbohydrate metabolism and controls blood sugar—providing energy
- Produces bile—necessary for the emulsion and absorption of fats
- Makes and breaks down hormones—needed throughout the body
- Detoxifies internal and environmental toxins—necessary for survival
- Filters everything in the blood—nutrients, food, drugs, toxins, and alcohol
- Contains cells, called Kuppfer cells, which are part of the immune system—they tell the body about toxins in the liver

The liver's biggest and toughest job is detoxification, especially considering the enormous amount of material that assaults us on a daily basis. Try to imagine for a

moment all the hundreds of chemicals and toxins floating through the blood waiting for cleansing and detoxification. It's like a line of hundreds of dirty campers
waiting for the only shower in the campground. Yet
these amazing livers of ours somehow manage to keep
up the process. Nevertheless, the constant job of trying
to detoxify all we put into our bodies can eventually
overwhelm it, leading to health problems.

There are several hundred problems related to liver
weakness. (See the "Symptoms of Liver Dysfunction" on
page 168 for a list conditions.)

Kidneys: The Water-Filtration System
The kidneys are so important that we have two of
them (some people are even born with three), although
people are able to survive with just one. They are shaped
like an ear and are purplish brown in color, weighing
about five ounces each, and measuring about four to
five inches long, three inches wide, and about one inch
thick. They are situated at the back of the abdominal
cavity, one on each side of the spine. The kidneys are
made up of microscopic nephrons that are responsible
for their functional and structural aspects and do most
of their major work.

The outer portion of the kidney is called the cortex.
It consists of capillary beds that filter the blood going
to the nephrons that are located in the inner part of the

kidneys. This is where filtration and reabsorption take place. The urine is formed inside the nephrons.

After the kidneys filter the blood, they return most of the water and many of the dissolved substances back to the bloodstream. What's left is called the urine, which passes through the ureters (tubular structures), then to the urinary bladder for storage, and finally through the urethra for elimination from the body.

Functions of the Kidneys

- Elimination of metabolic and toxic wastes
- Formation of urine from blood plasma
- Regulation of blood volume and blood pressure
- Regulation of ion levels in the blood
- Regulation of pH in the blood

The kidneys help excrete toxins by forming urine. Some of these waste products, including ammonia and urea from the breakdown of amino acids, are the result of metabolism and are greatly increased with the consumption of excess animal products. Additional waste products include bilirubin from the breakdown of hemoglobin from the blood; creatinine from the breakdown of creatine phosphate in muscle fibers; and uric acid from the breakdown of nucleic acids. Also, many of the essential ions such as sodium, chloride, sulfate, phosphate, and hydrogen tend to accumulate in excess of the body's needs and must be eliminated. In addition, the kidneys also excrete wastes from drugs, environmental toxins, and toxic substances from food and drink.

Kidneys are particularly sensitive to acidic wastes from such products as coffee, tea, soda pop, chocolate, and alcohol. The overconsumption of acidic products can lead to kidney distress and may be felt as pain in the lower back. Overconsumption of dairy products can lead to kidney stones, which are an accumulation of mineral salts combined mostly with calcium. The kidneys must handle all the excess toxicity that results when the liver and bowels are overwhelmed. The overconsumption of sugar and refined grains, salt, excess protein from animal products, and processed foods all put an additional burden on these organs.

THE LUNGS AND RESPIRATORY SYSTEM: THE AIR-FILTRATION SYSTEM

The respiratory system is comprised of the nose, pharynx, larynx, trachea, bronchi, and lungs. We have a set of lungs that are situated in what's called the thoracic cavity, or chest. They are cone-shaped, spongy organs that are separated from each other by the heart. The right lung is thicker and broader than the left, as well as slightly shorter because the liver is on this side extending up into the diaphragm.

The lungs are considered one of the five major organs of elimination. Their function is to breathe in oxygen, hydrogen, nitrogen, and carbon from the air and process it by extracting what the body needs for fuel. Without oxygen the cells of our bodies cannot produce energy from the food we eat. This process is called cellular respiration. It involves the reaction of glucose from the breakdown of our food in the presence of oxygen, which then produces energy, with carbon dioxide as an end product. This cellular respiration occurs in each of the cells of our bodies. The lungs then expel carbon dioxide gas, along with some of the toxic waste processed by the body.

Inhaled oxygen and other gases are exchanged through small sacs called alveoli; then they move into the pulmonary capillaries of the lungs where they are sent to the heart, which pumps them to every cell in the body. The waste products of cellular respiration are then picked up and sent back to the lungs for exhalation. Along the way these expelled gases act as a filter for other toxins that we inhale, such as dust, chemicals, and gases. They are then picked up by the capillaries of the lymphatic system and the blood and are sent to the lungs to be exhaled. Other toxic substances are trapped by mucus in the lungs and are subsequently coughed up and spit out with the mucus.

THE SKIN: THE CLEAN-UP CREW

Sometimes referred to as the third lung, the skin covers the entire surface area of our body, making it the largest organ of elimination. It is technically known as an organ because all of its tissues are structurally connected and it performs specific functions that benefit the entire body. One of these functions is to assist all the other organs of elimination in the process of detoxification, as well as acting as a barrier to prevent foreign or toxic substances from entering.

The Five Major Functions of the Skin

- Protection from toxins, bacteria, dehydration, and UV rays
- Excretion of wastes, water, salt, and organic compounds
- Maintenance of body temperature
- Perception of stimuli
- Synthesis of vitamin D

Due to its large surface area, the skin can eliminate through its pores as much waste as the bowels, kidneys, and lungs. This elimination is in the form of acidic toxins, gases, and mucus. If the colon, kidneys, or liver are backed up with toxic overload, the skin has to eliminate a larger part of the waste. If you are experiencing rashes, pimples, boils, acne, or abscesses, this indicates that your other organs of elimination are unable to keep up with detoxification. As you detoxify, you may have skin eruptions, so don't be alarmed. Your body is working to get rid of toxins as fast as possible; these conditions will soon clear up.

THE SUPPORTING CHANNELS
OF DETOXIFICATION

The gallbladder, lymphatic system, and blood support the work of the primary organs of elimination.

The Gallbladder: The Storage Tank

The gallbladder is a small pear-shaped organ that is located just under the right lobe of the liver. It's important in supporting the liver in eliminating toxins. The liver secretes toxins in a water-soluble form into the blood to either be excreted by the kidneys or by the colon. It's transported from the gallbladder by bile, which is a carrier substance whereby many toxins are expelled from the body. A type of "holding tank" for the bile, the gallbladder stores and concentrates bile that is made by the liver until it's needed by the small intestine.

Bile is made up of bile acids, salts, cholesterol, and electrolytes. It aids in digestion of fats. It's an alkaline substance that neutralizes stomach acid as the food comes out of the stomach and heads for the small intestine. In the meanwhile, the gallbladder stores bile until it gets a signal to contract and release it. In the gallbladder, water and minerals are absorbed from the bile, and it becomes darker in color, which produces a brown-colored stool. A light brown, walnut-colored stool is a sign that the bile is a good quality.

Lymphatic System: The Transport System

The lymphatic system is an arrangement of thin tubes that runs throughout the body called lymph vessels and lymph nodes. They branch throughout the body like the arteries except that they carry a colorless liquid called lymph — a clear fluid that circulates around the body tissues and contains a high number of lymphocytes (white blood cells). Plasma leaks out of the capillaries to surround and bathe the body tissues. This then drains into the lymph vessels. The lymphatic system also includes other organs — the spleen, thymus, tonsils, and adenoids.

The Lymphatic System Has Several Jobs

- Draining fluid back into the bloodstream from the tissues
- Filtering lymph
- Filtering the blood
- Fighting infections

The lymphatic system acts like a feeding station and drainage system for the cells of our body in that it carries nourishment to the cells and transports away some of the waste. Our cells are a bit like babies: They eat, produce energy, excrete waste, and depend on us for their care. The cells are nourished by oxygen and nutrients from the blood, they metabolize these raw materials to generate energy, and then they dump the waste products out. The lymph system picks up some of the waste where lymph nodes and other lymphatic organs filter the lymph to remove microorganisms and other foreign particles and lymphocytes destroy invading organisms.

Interstitial fluid is a watery substance that surrounds every cell in the body. It's the actual terrain that bathes the cells and picks up waste. It's particularly important to keep this fluid on the alkaline side by eating an alkaline-rich diet.

The lymphatic system is intimately connected to the immune system, and carries out four major functions:

1. Draining excess interstitial fluid
2. Helping to maintain proper fluid balance
3. Transporting dietary lipids to the blood — fats and fat-soluble vitamins (A, D, E, and K) that are absorbed by the intestinal tract are transported to the blood
4. Carrying out immune responses — lymphatic tissue initiates highly specific responses directed against particular microbes or abnormal cells

It's important to keep in mind that the lymphatic system does not have an active pump like the heart, but is instead moved by the skeletal respiratory pumps. Here's how it works: The skeletal muscles push against the lymphatic vessels squeezing them in a type of "milking action." The respiratory system causes pressure changes that occur during inhalation—lymph flows from the abdominal region, where pressure is higher, to the chest area, where it is lower.

The health of the lymphatic system is tied to the health of the liver. If the liver is not properly detoxifying waste, there will be more toxins entering the lymph. It's therefore important to cleanse and detoxify the liver periodically, which will assist the entire lymphatic system in its important work of carrying toxicity out of the body.

Blood: The River of Life

Blood is called our "river of life" for good reason; it brings life-giving nutrients like oxygen, vitamins, and minerals to the trillions of cells in our bodies, then carries waste to the organs of elimination. Blood is actively pumped throughout the body by the heart, unlike the lymph, which is a passive transport system.

Functions of Blood

- Regulation of pH—acidity or alkalinity (blood must be maintained at about 7.35–7.45 on the pH scale)
- Regulation of body temperature—normal is approximately 98.6
- Regulation of the water content of cells
- Transportation of oxygen to the cells from the lungs
- Transportation of carbon dioxide to the lungs
- Transportation of waste products from the cells to the liver, kidneys, lungs, and sweat glands to be expelled

Cleanse and Renew

Cleansing each of the organs of elimination is crucial if we want to have abundant health. We have seen the many ways toxins can accumulate in our organs of elimination. It's the accumulation of these toxins that keep many people in a place of "dis-ease" where they often feel sick and tired. To prevent illness and enjoy optimal health, it's imperative to get rid of the buildup of waste throughout the body by removing toxins, drug residues, heavy metals, acid, parasites, fungus, yeasts, and other pathogens. As you detoxify your organs and systems of elimination you'll begin to feel better, perhaps better than you've felt in years. Cleansing will give you an amazing sense of well-being, energy, and life! Plus, it will help you prevent disease. Your reward will be a life of abundant health and the energy to fulfill your purpose.

The programs that follow have worked for me and for countless numbers of people whom I've worked with through the years. The elimination of wastes and toxins will facilitate weight loss, oftentimes where nothing else may have worked. People often exclaim that their excess weight just melted away! And cellulite, which is trapped toxins, water, and fat cells, usually improves or goes away completely.

Adding a detoxification program can dramatically change your health and give you a more youthful appearance. I encourage you to stick with these cleansing programs until you have systematically detoxed each major organ or system in your body. You will be rewarded with high-level wellness.

Summary of Detoxing for Life

Step 1: Eat whole, alkalizing, organic, non-GMO foods; remove as many sources of toxicity as possible; drink plenty of purified water, and eat 50 to 75 percent of your food raw.

Step 2: Add fresh vegetable juices to your diet at least once or twice a day.

Step 3: Complete a one- to three-day juice fast.

Step 4: Complete the colon, liver and gallbladder, and/or kidney cleanse programs.

CHAPTER FIVE

Colon Cleansing for Vibrant Health

While colon cleansing is far from a sexy subject, the results it achieves are truly exciting. It's one of the most effective keys for weight loss and great health.

Whether you call it the large intestine, bowel, or colon, the reality is that for a lot of us, it's congested. A thorough colon cleansing is a great way to boost your energy and vitality and overcome some common symptoms of ill health such as poor digestion, constipation, acid reflux, stomach pain, irritable bowel syndrome, *Candida albicans*, gas, bloating, protruding belly, headaches, and low energy. And if you want to lose weight quickly and easily, it's crucial to cleanse the intestinal tract.

Colon cleansing is one of the most important steps —

and usually the most overlooked — when it comes to losing weight, reshaping the body, flattening the abdomen, improving digestion and elimination, and restoring health. The problem is that we can't properly digest and eliminate food and substances we ingest when the colon is congested. The more congested it is, the more waste in the form of old fecal matter and mucus can lodge in the lining. People can end up carrying around pounds of this stuff. Not only does this interfere with the normal two to three bowel movements per day needed for good health, it interferes with nutrient absorption from our food and supplements.

Combining colon cleansing with a good weight-loss diet, such as *The Coconut Diet* (our program for effective weight loss), can help you trim your waistline faster and more completely than any diet by itself. A stomach that protrudes may not be just from fat; it can also be the result of intestinal waste buildup. When the entire intestinal tract is cleansed, the stomach often flattens. The colon can also function better, eliminating wastes quicker, which greatly facilitates weight loss and boosts health. And nutrient absorption is improved so your body is better fed. As a result, cravings usually diminish or disappear, making it easier to stick with your healthy lifestyle program.

It's always a good idea to begin a detox with a thorough cleansing of the bowel before you move on to other organs. When your body detoxifies, it dislodges poisons and toxins that have built up in cells and tissues. Your body will pull toxins out of all their hiding places. These wastes are then deposited in the colon for rapid elimination, but if it's congested with old fecal matter, then the toxins can't skip on out as easily. They'll just sit around and get reabsorbed back into the bloodstream. And you could experience more headaches, weakness, fevers, chills, nausea, skin eruptions, and other detox symptoms.

The Root of Many Health Problems

A congested colon is at the root of numerous health problems. Some natural healing professionals believe it's the principal cause of nearly every disease. Considering we spend seven hundred to eight hundred million dollars a year in this country on laxatives, it's fair to say that many Americans have sluggish, constipated bowels. Dr. Bernard Jensen was a pioneering chiropractor and nutritionist who began his career in 1929 writing about proper bowel management. His books are still considered classics in the field of detoxification. Dr. Jensen states that "In the fifty years I've spent helping people to overcome illness, disability and disease, it has become crystal clear that poor bowel management lies at the root of most people's health problems."

Clogging Versus Cleansing Foods

CLOGGING (COLON UNFRIENDLY)	CLEANSING (COLON FRIENDLY)
• Refined flour products (e.g., bread, pasta, pizza dough, bagels) • Cheese • Other dairy products • Meat • Trans fats • Sweet treats and desserts • Snack foods (potato chips, corn chips, bagel chips, cheese puffs, etc.) • Fast foods (French fries, burgers, tacos, deep-fried foods)	• Vegetables (especially high water content) • Fresh vegetable juices • Fresh whole fruit • Whole grains (e.g., brown rice, quinoa, barley) • Legumes (beans, split peas, lentils) • Flaxseeds (ground) • Most nuts (soaked in water or ground are best) • Fresh herbs (e.g., parsley, cilantro, basil) • Filtered or purified water • Herbal teas • Fiber supplements

What Happens When the Colon Doesn't Work Efficiently?

The following points will help you better understand what is going on in the intestinal tract when it's not functioning well:

- The feces becomes dehydrated and compacted in the colon, leading to constipation, which many health professionals believe contributes to disease.
- Old fecal matter and sticky mucus can become lodged or stuck to the sides of the intestinal tract, which leads to an irritation of the lining of the colon.

- Pathogenic organisms like bacteria, viruses, parasites, and yeasts such as *Candida albicans* are able to proliferate in a toxic colon. These pathogens excrete waste material in the form of toxic enzymes, acids, and gases that cause inflammation and eventual degradation of the intestinal walls.
- When the feces are moving too slowly through the bowel, the toxins have more time to penetrate the bowel wall and move into the bloodstream.
- Recirculating toxins cause weakness in tissues and organs throughout the body.
- Toxins accumulate in our cells, tissues, blood, and organs such as the colon, liver, and brain and stay there, causing numerous health problems.
- The immune system becomes overwhelmed with the toxic overload as white blood cells take up toxic debris. This leaves us vulnerable to a host of diseases.

Symptoms of a Toxic Colon

Digestive health can suffer as a result of toxic overload in the colon and can lead to seemingly unrelated problems like skin conditions, joint pain, sinus problems, varicose veins, forgetfulness, and irritability, to name just a few. A malfunctioning colon is at the root of hundreds of illnesses and diseases.

Often people think their health concern has nothing

to do with the colon because it is manifested somewhere else in the body. For example, an impacted colon can press against nerves and cause back pain, sciatica, and leg pain, since it's in close proximity to the nerves from the spine or an impacted colon can release toxins that travel to other parts of the body causing headaches and sinus infections.

Symptoms of a Toxic Colon

The following symptoms are often associated with a congested colon. They indicate the need to detoxify or cleanse your bowel:

- Chronic constipation
- Gas and bloating
- Diarrhea
- Weight gain and inability to lose weight
- Low energy or fatigue
- Impaired digestion
- Stomach pain
- Irritable bowel syndrome (IBS)
- Leaky gut syndrome
- Acid reflux or heartburn (GERD)
- Diverticulitis
- Crohn's disease
- Swollen or protruding belly
- *Candida albicans* (yeast infection)
- Parasites
- Food allergies
- Gluten sensitivity
- Lactose intolerance
- Hemorrhoids
- Irritability, mood swings
- Foul-smelling stools or gas
- Frequent colds
- Chronic headaches
- Rashes, skin eruptions
- Colon cancer

Common Problems of the Colon

Following are common bowel problems that plague millions of Americans. These conditions can be greatly improved with a colon detoxification program.

CONSTIPATION

Constipation refers to the difficulty or infrequency in passing stools. Constipation can undermine the health of the whole body, affecting digestion, preventing a clearing of toxins, lowering energy levels, and hindering efficient absorption of nutrients.

Poor diet is a major contributor to constipation, as is poor liver function, parasites, *Candida albicans*, and low thyroid function, along with nutrient deficiencies such as magnesium and vitamin C. Food allergies and sensitivities can also be contributing factors. Too much dairy and refined grains can be quite constipating. And stress has an adverse effect.

The treatment of constipation includes adequate fiber, plenty of water, sufficient vitamin C and magnesium, improvement in thyroid health, exercise, and *Candida albicans* and parasite cleansing, along with colon and liver cleansing. When you cleanse the intestinal tract, constipation is usually alleviated and weight loss becomes easier. Drinking fresh vegetable juices can also be very helpful, since they supply a good source of soluble fiber, which is very beneficial to the colon.

COLON CANCER

Colon cancer, or colorectal cancer, involves cancerous growths in the colon, rectum, or appendix. More people die each year from colorectal cancer than from breast cancer and AIDS combined. After lung cancer, it is the leading cause of death from cancer in both men and women. It's the third most diagnosed cancer in the United States and Canada (excluding skin cancer). Only lung and breast cancer in women, and lung and prostate cancer in men are diagnosed more frequently.

Studies show that a diet high in red meat and low in vegetables, fruit, and other high-fiber foods contributes to an increased risk of colon cancer. The best preventive program is one that includes reducing clogging foods, eating more cleansing foods, drinking more water, exercising, and completing periodic colon cleansing, along with periodic preventive testing for those at high risk or over fifty.

DIVERTICULOSIS OR DIVERTICULAR DISEASE

The latest statistics reveal that the number of Americans who suffer from diverticulosis is increasing. The National Institute of Diabetes and Digestive and Kidney Diseases (NIDDK) reported that 10 percent of Americans over forty have diverticulosis. By age sixty the figure jumps to 50 percent. The good news is that proper care of the colon can prevent this condition or keep it from developing into the more serious form known as diverticulitis.

Diverticulosis is a condition that results when small pouches called diverticula form in the colon. These pouches bulge outward through weak spots in the colon wall. If they become infected, the condition is called diverticulitis. Diverticular disease is believed to be caused principally by a low-fiber diet that leads to constipation. The resulting pressure on the colon wall causes a diverticula to form. It's interesting to note that diverticular disease was not even observed in the United States until the early part of the 1900s when low-fiber, processed foods were first introduced into the American diet.

Contributors to Poor Colon Health

In addition to poor diet, lack of exercise, insufficient fiber, and not drinking enough water, there are a number of other factors that contribute to poor colon health, including stress, an imbalance of good and bad bacteria, inadequate chewing of food, overeating, and improper food combining.

Toxic emotions such as fear, stress, worry, and anxiety take a particular toll on the digestive system. The autonomic nervous system controls all unconscious activity in the body, including control of the digestive system. When it's stressed, the nervous system diverts energy away from the digestive organs and routes it to the musculo-skeletal system to mobilize us for action in what is known as the "flight or fight" response. During this stress reaction, the intestines and kidneys slow down so the body can run away or fight the enemy. The problem with our fast-paced lifestyles is that we perceive threat on a continuous basis, and our digestive system suffers continually. Stress also decreases saliva flow and lowers the output of digestive enzymes and hydrochloric acid. A stressful lifestyle results in impaired digestion and decreased bowel function. To help your digestive health, it's best not to eat when emotionally upset, angry, or worried until you can calm down and let your body return to a state of balance.

IMBALANCE OF GOOD AND BAD BACTERIA

A healthy intestinal tract has a complex ecology of friendly, neutral, and unfriendly (pathogenic) bacteria. An overgrowth of unfriendly bacteria, yeasts, and parasites can disrupt the delicate balance of the entire gastrointestinal tract. This overgrowth eventually leads to inflammation in the sensitive mucus lining, which then interferes with the proper assimilation of nutrients.

The contributing factors to imbalanced intestinal flora include a diet that is high in animal fats, trans fats, processed foods, low-fiber foods, sugar, coffee, tea, and alcohol, as well as overuse of antibiotics, over-the-counter drugs like acetaminophen and aspirin (NSAIDs), plus a diet that lacks essential nutrients. Antibiotics are particularly damaging to this delicate balance because they not only kill the bacteria they were prescribed for, they destroy friendly bacteria in the colon. The good bacteria have many beneficial functions, such as converting certain raw materials into much-needed nutrients. They're also responsible for keeping pathogenic bacteria and yeast that live in the colon in check. Once this delicate balance is disrupted, the unfriendly bacteria begin to outnumber the good, which causes more toxins to be released. Additionally, yeasts rapidly proliferate, causing more problems because candida releases numerous toxins into the body, including acetaldehyde and ethyl alcohol.

A typical American diet that is high in bad fat and refined carbs and low in fiber has a tendency to stick to the inner walls of the intestinal tract, and results in an impacted layer developing in the intestines. This condition eventually leads to a buildup of mucus, which decreases the available binding sites for the good bacteria. Removing this toxic-laden mucus layer through colon cleansing enables the friendly bacteria to attach to the intestinal walls again and helps restore the balance of intestinal flora. Use of a good probiotic formula will reintroduce friendly bacteria such as *Lactobacillus acidophilus* and *Lactobacillus bifidus* into the colon.

Simple Tips for Optimal Digestion

Are you one of those busy people who eat meals on the run? Many people get so hurried with their busy schedules that they grab something quick and easy, barely chew it, and then wash it down with a big gulp of soda pop, iced tea, or water. If this describes you, you may have noticed that your digestion is not as good as it used to be. Most of us can get away with this to some degree when we're young, but the older we get, the more our digestion becomes challenged by a hurried lifestyle. One of the best ways to help your digestion improve is to slow down, take a few breaths, say a thanksgiving for your food, and slowly begin chewing thoroughly. Instead of thinking "fast food," start thinking in terms of "slow food" eating. Set aside enough time in your schedule to do nothing but eat, preferably enjoying your food with family and friends as often as possible, the way many Europeans do.

Digestion actually begins in the mouth. First we chew our food, breaking it down into smaller and smaller particles. As we chew, saliva mixes with the food and starts the process of digestion. Saliva contains the enzymes ptyalin and amylase that begin digestion of the carbohydrates in vegetables, fruit, starches, and sugars in the mouth. Other enzymes act on any bacteria that might be in the food, thereby providing the first line of defense against foreign invaders. Not taking the time to properly chew your food interferes with this initial digestion process and can lead to many problems down the line such as indigestion, acid reflux, leaky gut syndrome, and constipation.

Your mother was right when she said, "Chew, chew, chew your food!" You need to chew each mouthful at least twenty to thirty times before you swallow it. Insufficient chewing puts stress on the digestive system because food particles that are not broken down well enter the intestines, where they can produce toxic metabolites that leak through the membranes in the intestines.

Limit the amount of water you drink with meals, especially ice-cold liquids, because they can interfere with proper digestion. Too much liquid with meals dilutes the digestive enzymes in the mouth and the stomach, so the food is not properly digested, leading to many of the problems we've been discussing. The stomach contains hydrochloric acid that acts on proteins, denaturing them and preparing them for the next stage of digestion. The stomach also contains a protein-digesting enzyme called pepsin and a fat-digesting enzyme known as lipase. Drinking too much liquid with your meals makes it difficult for these enzymes to work efficiently, so food enters the intestines in a partially undigested state. Try to drink no more than four ounces of liquid with your meals, preferably at room temperature. The approach is to stop drinking lots of liquids about half an hour before meals and then resume at least a half hour after.

Overeating

In these days of supersize meals, most people have become accustomed to eating far too much food. Americans have been programmed by the food industry to eat, eat, eat, but the sad news is that overeating causes more health problems than just about anything else. Even eating too much healthy food puts a strain on the digestive system and can lead to problems like obesity, high blood pressure, heart disease, acid reflux, and constipation.

Many studies have shown that people who habitually undereat live longer and are healthier than their overeating counterparts. Calorie restriction helps improve health and slow the aging process. Smaller portions support digestive health. We can be particularly watchful when eating out. For example, instead of heaping food on our plate from a buffet, we can choose a reasonable serving. In restaurants that serve large portions, we can share a dinner with a friend or ask for a take-home carton. One easy rule of thumb is to eat only half as much as you are accustomed to. You'll be surprised at how quickly your body adapts to smaller portions. And your waistline will reap a big reward!

Improper Food Combining

There are many theories about how to combine food for maximum digestive health, and a certain amount of disagreement exists among health practitioners. Nevertheless, there are a few standards that almost everyone agrees on. The most important rule is not to mix heavy protein foods like meat with starchy carbohydrates such as potatoes or refined carbohydrates like bread and pasta. This teaching challenges the tradition of hamburgers and sandwiches, or meat and potatoes that are so popular in our culture. This is not to say that you can't ever have such a meal again, but work on having them less often. The problem is that proteins require different digestive enzymes than carbohydrates. If you have digestive challenges, try eating your protein with only vegetables, and especially include some high-water-content foods like green leafy vegetables. A big salad, a steamed vegetable, and a small piece of free-range poultry or fish are an ideal alternative to meat, potatoes, and bread. If you choose to have a meal of grains rather than protein, use whole grains like rice, quinoa (pronounced *keen-wa*), millet, or spelt combined with lightly steamed vegetables and a big salad. This way of eating is not only more conducive to good digestive health, but is the way to maintain a good alkaline balance — one of the pillars of a healthy eating program.

The Goal of the Colon-Cleansing Program

Completing a colon cleanse will help you improve digestion and colon health. By eliminating waste that's stuck in the large intestine, you create a better environment for evacuation. Also, colon cleansing increases the colon's ability to absorb essential nutrients and water. The results will be a better-nourished body.

"What is a normal bowel movement?" people frequently ask. It's surprising how many people think *normal* is to have one bowel movement every other day, or even less often. For some, it's once a week. Health researchers have studied people who live in nonindustrialized, rural communities, who eat a simple, natural, whole foods diet and get a moderate amount of exercise. They've determined that these people set the standard for a healthy colon. You might be surprised to learn that they will have a bowel movement within about a half hour after eating a meal, which means that their bowels move two to three times a day. Two to three times a day should be our goal. And yes, it's possible to reach this goal once the colon is cleansed and restored to health.

Another question people frequently ask is "What does a healthy bowel movement look like?" Healthy feces will be walnut brown in color, will appear soft and unformed, with about the consistency of peanut butter, and will float for a moment before slowly sinking as it begins to break up. It will not be hard, dark in color, pencil thin, or a series of hard pellets. By this definition, there aren't too many people in America who can report that their colons are working efficiently most of the time.

The goal in the colon-cleansing program is to remedy poor colon health by restoring normal muscle movement in the intestines (peristalsis) so the waste that is inhibiting digestion and assimilation can be removed. The colon cleanse program will require some time and effort for a week or two, but the rewards are well worth it. If we cooperate with our bodies, and cleanse our colon, it will heal and function normally again.

The Colon-Detoxification Program

A thorough detoxification program includes these six important steps:

1. Reduce exposure to toxins—environmental or from processed foods.
2. Eat a health-building diet—with plenty of vegetables and fresh vegetable juices.
3. Eliminate coffee, alcohol, nicotine, and over-the-counter medications.
4. Exercise—sweat to eliminate toxins.
5. Drink plenty of water to flush toxins.
6. Detoxify your colon.

The Colon-Cleanse Program

During the colon-cleanse program, you can eat two to three meals a day, but they should be light and healthy, mostly raw with plenty of raw vegetables, vegetable juices, and some low-sugar fruit such as berries or green apples. During the colon cleanse you will be eating lots of colon-cleansing, alkaline foods like high-water-content green leafy vegetables and brightly colored vegetables, plenty of fresh vegetable juices, vegetable smoothies, fresh whole fruit, and ground raw seeds and nuts. The cleanse works best when you avoid heavy animal foods like meats, cheese, and other dairy products and processed grains such as bread and pasta. You can have an egg or a little fish, but I recommend limiting them as much as possible for maximum colon cleansing. You can have any of the colon-friendly foods listed in the box on page 133, but limit whole grains and legumes to a small amount once a day. You are encouraged to eat lighter, smaller portions of everything except raw vegetables. Also, make sure you drink plenty of purified water to assist the cleansing process.

Stick with the Colon Cleanse as long as it takes to complete the job. If you have never tried a colon cleanse, it will probably take two weeks, possibly more, to complete. It's rare that the colon can be cleansed in just one week the first time. If you have completed colon cleanses in the past on a regular basis, then one week will probably work well. The more diligent you are about sticking to mostly raw foods (50 to 75 percent) and drinking plenty of vegetable juices, the more quickly you can complete the program. For those who are transitioning to more alkaline, colon-friendly fare, continue adding fresh raw foods and juices as much as possible, and stay with the program as outlined. This is not a race to the finish, but a process of change to help your body in its detoxification of this important organ of elimination.

Follow the sample menu guidelines below and remember, this is only for a week or two, not forever. If two weeks of colon cleansing do not get your bowels working properly, then return to step one of healthy eating for a week or two, and try another colon cleanse later.

MENU PLAN

Upon Rising
   7:00 A.M. Fiber Shake (see suggestions on page 151)*

Breakfast — 8:00 A.M.
   Choose one of the following:

   1. Awesome Green Smoothie with almonds, or
   2. Avocado and sliced tomatoes, or
   3. One of the vegetable juice recipes in chapter ten

   9:00 A.M. Probiotic
   10:00 A.M. Fresh vegetable juice such as the Colon
       Cleanse Cocktail or any juice recipe
   11:00 A.M. Fiber Shake

*You'll need to purchase a good fiber product designed for colon cleansing.

Lunch — 12:00 Noon

Choose one of the following:

1. Large mixed vegetable salad and a cup of raw soup (see recipes starting on page 301)

2. Large mixed vegetable salad with avocado (be creative and add lots of different vegetables) with ½ cup cooked brown rice (or other whole grains like quinoa or millet)

3. Chopped hearty vegetable salad — bite-size pieces of broccoli, cauliflower, red and green pepper, celery, cucumber, radishes, tomato, yellow squash, and zucchini; add some sprouted alfalfa or sunflower seeds, cilantro, or parsley for variety

Salad dressing favorite: 1/2 cup extra-virgin olive oil, 3 tablespoons Bragg Liquid Aminos* (from health food store), 3 tablespoons lemon juice, 3 tablespoons water. Shake together in a glass container and add fresh minced garlic or ground garlic to taste, and herbs of choice.

---

*The Bragg Liquid Aminos tastes similar to soy sauce (but is not a soy product); it's salty, so you may want to start with a small amount. You can also use just olive oil and lemon juice. Olive oil is very cleansing, as is lemon juice. Avoid commercial salad dressings, especially during cleansing.

Afternoon

> 3:00 P.M. Fiber Shake
>
> 4:00 P.M. If hungry, choose a juice or smoothie recipe
> or low-sugar fruit like berries or a green apple

Dinner — 6:00 P.M.

> Prepare a dinner that follows the healthy guidelines.
> Use one of the lunch suggestions, or be creative
> with vegetable dishes. Be sure to include plenty of
> raw vegetables such as a salad, sliced tomatoes, veg-
> etable sticks, or lightly steamed vegetables like broc-
> coli, asparagus, Brussels sprouts, carrots, and onions.
> You may add 1 or 2 ounces of chicken, turkey, or fish,
> if you really have to have more protein, but remem-
> ber that animal products are clogging as opposed
> to cleansing, so it's best if you can omit them. Your
> cleanse will proceed more quickly if you skip all
> animal protein. You will not lose muscle mass while
> forgoing animal protein for a week or two.

After Dinner

> Herbal cleanse formula. Take according to directions,
> usually one or two capsules is sufficient (see Resources
> Guide). (Herbal colon cleanse products must be pur-
> chased. Use according to manufacturer's directions.)
>
> 8:00 P.M. Herbal tea and probiotic
> 9:00 P.M. Fiber Shake

DURING THE CLEANSE

During the cleanse you will have four fiber shakes a day, plus an herbal cleaning formula at least once, usually after dinner. Continue to drink plenty of water between meals, aiming for two to two and a half quarts per day (there's four eight-ounce glasses per quart, so that's eight to ten glasses a day). Also, you may drink herbal tea throughout the day and count it toward your water quota. You can sweeten drinks with a little stevia, but don't use sugar or honey. Earlier in the day it's fine to have one or two cups of green tea or white tea, both of which contain some caffeine, though not as much as coffee, but avoid them later in the day or if you tend toward low blood sugar or poor adrenal function.

Fiber Shake

You'll want to eat a high-fiber diet during this program, as well as on your maintenance program, and you'll also add additional fiber as part of the cleanse in order to facilitate the movement of impacted waste from the colon. The fiber acts like a broom to sweep the walls of the colon, and like sponges to soak up toxins and waste material so they can be eliminated.

The colon cleanse products used should include flax fiber, or ground flaxseeds, bentonite clay, and a small amount of ground psyllium husks or seeds. Other good fibers are apple or citrus pectin and guar gum. Adding activated charcoal helps to absorb even more of the toxins as they are released.

There are a number of products available, or you can mix your own. Many commercial products principally contain psyllium husks or seeds, which in large amounts can cause bloating or constipation in some people and may be too drying for your colon. But a small amount mixed with other fiber usually works quite well. I don't recommend wheat bran since so many people are sensitive to wheat; alternatives include oat bran and rice bran. Other possibilities include acacia gum and microcrystalline cellulose. Read labels carefully before purchasing a product (see Resources Guide).

HOMEMADE FIBER BLEND

Most of the products listed here are available in your local health food store or natural foods store. You may also want to purchase a seed grinder or an inexpensive small coffee grinder so you can grind your own flaxseeds.

1/2 cup flax fiber or ground flaxseeds
1/2 cup bentonite clay
2 tablespoons ground psyllium husks or seeds
2 tablespoons activated charcoal (optional)
2–3 tablespoons apple or citrus pectin (optional)

Mix all these dry ingredients together in a plastic container or glass jar and refrigerate.

For your fiber shake mix one to one and a half large tablespoons of this mixture together in eight ounces of water or vegetable juice and shake well. For added flavor you can add a teaspoon of lemon or lime juice or unsweetened cranberry juice concentrate to the water.

Cleansing Herbs and Supplements

There are many commercial colon-cleansing products available that make use of various herbs and nutrients that are beneficial for moving the bowels. You will want to choose a product that works well for you. The goal is to get your bowels moving two to three times a day and to gently and naturally cleanse the walls of the colon to remove impacted material and eliminate stored toxins. Magnesium is an excellent mineral that helps alleviate constipation by drawing water into the intestines, causing the feces to soften. Herbs that help in colon cleansing include slippery elm bark, marshmallow root, peppermint leaf, coriander, gentian, cinnamon, rhubarb root, papaya, cayenne, spearmint, garlic, fennel, and gingerroot. Cascara sagrada and senna are stimulant herbs with a laxative effect; they can be too harsh for some people. They can be quite beneficial during a colon cleanse, but should not be used long term as they can create dependence. Some people are so constipated that they need a formula that includes one or both, along with more soothing herbs like slippery elm, marshmallow root, and peppermint (see Resources Guide).

THE COLON CLEANSE JUICE COCKTAIL

1 cucumber, peeled if not
organic
1 handful spinach,
washed

1 handful parsley, washed
1 stalk celery, washed
1/4 to 1/2 medium lemon,
peeled

Cut the cucumber in half or the size that will fit your juicer feed tube. Bunch up the spinach and parsley and push through the juicer with the cucumber, celery, and lemon.

AWESOME GREEN SMOOTHIE

1 small to medium
cucumber, peeled if not
organic
2 cups spinach, washed
1 medium to large
avocado, peeled with
seed removed

1 tablespoon virgin
coconut oil (optional)
Juice from one lime or
lemon
Stevia to sweeten
(optional)
Add a little water, if needed

Cut the cucumber into chunks, put in blender and process until smooth. Add spinach and blend until smooth. Cut the avocado into chunks, add to blender along with coconut oil and the remaining ingredients. Blend until smooth. Add water, as needed. Pour into bowls. Makes two servings. Or you can store the second serving in a container for use later in the day.

NOTE: This smoothie is good served with chopped or ground raw almonds that have been soaked overnight in the refrigerator for easy digestion and then dehydrated. All nuts can be digested better if they are first soaked in water. This releases enzyme inhibitors. You can dehydrate nuts in advance, and grind, then sprinkle on top of the smoothie.

Colon Detoxification Helpers

PROBIOTICS

As you cleanse, it's very important to restore healthy intestinal flora (bacteria) in the gut by taking what is known as a "probiotic" (beneficial bacteria) formula. Often, the body's beneficial bacteria have been depleted by the use of antibiotics, other medications, and years of poor eating habits. Probiotics also restore healthful bacteria after cleansing. Proper bacteria are essential for a strong immune system, assimilation of vitamins, proteins, fats, and carbohydrates; the manufacture of B vitamins; and to keep yeasts such as *Candida albicans* and parasites under control. (For recommendations, see Resources Guide.) Depending on the formula you choose as your probiotic, you may need to take probiotics more or less often than is recommended on the menu schedule.

COLONICS

Colon hydrotherapy, which is popularly known as a *colonic,* entails flushing the colon with water, usually by a professional colon therapist. Colon hydrotherapy is a safe, effective method of removing waste from the large intestine, without the use of drugs. Intestinal waste is softened and loosened by introducing pure, filtered, temperature-regulated water into the colon, which results in evacuation of waste. A colonic or two per week during the one to two weeks of colon cleansing is particularly beneficial in removing excess waste. It can also be helpful in facilitating weight loss.

If you're thinking, "No way would I consider this," it might be of interest to know that some of the most glamorous people we watch in the media have taken advantage of this health practice. It's been reported that Princess Diana was an avid fan of colonics, and it's rumored that numerous Hollywood stars regularly go for colonics. The reason partakers range from royalty to Hollywood stars to everyday people is that colonics help to reduce bloating and gas, flatten protruding tummies, facilitate weight loss, improve colon health, and beautify the skin. I've combined colonics with juice fasting and intestinal herbal cleansing several times a year for more than fifteen years, and on more than one occasion, I've experienced a two-pound weight loss after a colonic.

Toxins can build up on the intestinal wall just like plaque builds up on teeth. Can you imagine never having your teeth cleaned? Colon irrigation hydrates the colon and assists in the removal of built-up fecal matter, mucus, and toxins.

Although it might be disconcerting to the very shy, most practitioners will immediately make you feel relaxed, at ease, and safe. However, make sure the center you choose is clean and uses disposable hoses and tubes.

People who get colonics usually rave about the effects they experience, such as improved colon health, a flatter stomach, a clearing of the whites of their eyes, improvement in skin health and appearance, and a luminescence to their skin and hair. If you cannot find a colon therapist in your area, enemas are the next best thing.

THE ENEMA

Enemas have been used for centuries to maintain bowel health. They can be very beneficial in restoring regularity. It was common practice for past generations to use enemas to treat nearly every illness. During a colon cleanse, an enema is excellent for clearing out the debris that is being released from intestinal walls.

An enema entails infusing water into the colon through the anus. You can find enema bags in some drugstores (usually the independent stores). The easiest to use are those that look like a hot water bag. You simply fill the bag with about one quart of warm water —

filtered or distilled is best — then lie down on your left side, insert the end of the hose into your anus, making sure the clamp is on tightly so the water doesn't go all over the floor. If you'll remember from our discussion of the anatomy of the colon, the descending colon runs down the left side of the body. This is why it's best to lie down on the left side starting out. Reach behind for the clamp to release it and let the water run in until you start to feel full, then clamp it off for a moment. Unclamp and continue until all the water has drained into your colon. Relax and wait for a few minutes on your left side, then turn on your back for a couple of minutes to allow the water to go across your transverse colon. (Unless you just can't wait. Sometimes, in the beginning, this is hard to do.) Next you should turn onto your right side for a couple of minutes so the water can go into the ascending colon. After this you will want to evacuate all the water and waste. Take the time to let everything expel. Then relax, and stay close to the bathroom for another ten to fifteen minutes.

There are a number of substances that you can add to the water as infusions that can help facilitate the removal of toxic material. Wheatgrass juice is very beneficial because it contains so many healing nutrients and the chlorophyll is detoxifying. It can be made by adding 1 to 2 ounces of wheatgrass juice to 2 cups of warm water. Coffee enemas are sometimes used, but I don't recommend them because the caffeine is absorbed through the colon and acts as a liver stimulant. The simplest and easiest enema is just to use warm water.

Exercises to Facilitate Colon Cleansing

The benefits of exercise for overall health and wellness are undisputed. Exercise increases energy, helps you lose weight, increases muscle strength and tone, and helps in cardiovascular fitness. During cleansing, exercise assists in the elimination of toxins. Specific benefits during cleansing include the following:

- Increased blood flow so more oxygen reaches your cells and more toxins can be picked up
- Decreased stress and anxiety so the entire digestive system can work more efficiently
- Increased lymph flow, which is crucial for the removal of toxins and for increased immune function
- Increased sweating so toxins can be eliminated through the skin
- Increased rate of breathing to eliminate toxins through the lungs

Aerobic exercises are particularly beneficial during cleansing because they increase your heart rate over a sustained time, which boosts oxygen flow through the blood and into every cell in your body. Start with as much as you are able to do. If you aren't accustomed to exercise, work up to at least twenty to thirty minutes or more of sustained movement for maximum benefit at least three days a week; eventually increase to sixty minutes, for a minimum of three times per week. Examples of aerobic exercise include running, jogging, fast walking, swimming, bicycling, dancing, skating, step aerobics classes, or rebounding.

Rebounding is one of the best exercises you can do to assist your body during the process of detoxification. It's an exercise performed on a mini trampoline, which is appropriately called a rebounder. It's fun, easy to do, safe, and very effective. You can jump on it in the comfort of your own home — no need to pound the pavement, avoid cars, or put up with bad weather.

It's also a zero-impact aerobic exercise that improves blood circulation and increases the capacity of both the heart and lungs, plus it is one of the most effective exercises for moving the fluids of the lymphatic system, which carry waste products out of our bodies. Vigorous exercise such as rebounding can significantly increase lymph flow. Because lymph is totally dependent on physical exercise (or lymphatic drainage massage) to move, without adequate movement the lymph system cannot properly excrete toxic waste products, which then affects the cells, limiting their ability to efficiently absorb life-giving nutrients.

Exercise is very important for the lymphatic system because there is no active lymph pump to move it through the lymph vessels like our heart pumps blood through the blood vessels. The lymphatic system is passive, not active, and the vessels of the lymphatic system have valves that move it in one direction only. Therefore, active movement is required to keep the fluids moving. The main lymph vessels run up the legs, arms, and up the torso, so a vertical up-and-down movement is especially effective at pumping lymph through the vessels.

Regardless of what activity you do, the main point during a cleanse is to exert yourself enough to increase your breathing and break a sweat. The process of sweating greatly facilitates the removal of toxins, which will make your detoxing much easier and more effective. In addition to exercise, saunas, either infrared or regular, and/or hot soaking baths, especially in natural mineral springs, will induce sweating and facilitate the elimination of toxins.

Summary of Colon Detoxing

Step 1:   Eat whole, alkalizing foods, emphasizing organic, non-GMO foods. Remove as many sources of toxicity as possible, drink plenty of water, and eat 50–75 percent of your food raw

(Continued)

Step 2: Add fresh vegetable juices to your diet at least once or
twice a day

Step 3: Complete one to three days of juice fasting

Step 4: Colon-Detoxification Program

- Increase consumption of water, juice, and herbal tea to
  flush out toxins.
- Eat colon-cleansing foods and limit colon-clogging foods
  (see box page 133).
- Add a fiber shake four times during the day.
- Take an herbal cleansing formula one or more times
  daily (follow product directions).
- Take a colonic or an enema at least once or twice
  during the program.
- Add aerobic exercises to increase heart rate and
  induce sweating.
- Take saunas or hot baths during the cleanse to facilitate
  sweating.

CHAPTER SIX

Liver, Gallbladder, and Kidney Cleansing

If your washing machine was broken down, your drain was clogged, or your water heater was leaking, you'd get to work right away to make repairs. Your liver, gallbladder, and kidneys are far more important than any household appliance, yet they often get far less attention. Isn't it time to cleanse these hardworking organs and get them in good working condition again?

The detox programs that follow will help you cleanse the liver, gallbladder, and kidneys and assist them in functioning well so you can feel healthy, energetic, and really alive. It may seem strange to think that the liver, gallbladder, and kidneys have something to do with how you feel, but they do. Their health is key to your overall health. You'll never know just how good you can feel until you cleanse these organs of elimination. So let's get started with the Liver Detoxification Program.

Liver Detoxification

The liver is the largest and most complex internal organ in the human body. It performs hundreds of tasks every minute of every day, more than any other organ, including the brain. The brain processes information like a computer, but the liver processes physiological tasks like a busy work crew. It's constantly filtering, detoxifying, synthesizing, and processing a wide variety of substances. Without a healthy, well-functioning liver you can quickly become toxic, which leads to feeling tired, sick, and often depressed. You might notice your fingers and toes aren't as thin as they once were, because impaired liver function causes decreased serum albumen, which leads to edema swelling due to fluid accumulation in the tissues. Or maybe your hormones are out of whack because the liver metabolizes most hormones, and when it's not functioning well, hormone metabolism is off.

The liver is the main organ of detoxification in the body, filtering and cleansing approximately fifty gallons of blood every day. The liver acts much like a coffee filter in straining out harmful toxins and ammonia. They're removed from the blood and transformed before being eliminated through the bowels or the kidneys. The liver also processes the pollutants that we breathe in through our lungs or absorb through our skin. Whether toxins are from environmental pollution, processed or contaminated food, or are internally produced, they're all detoxified in the liver in a complex, two-step process known as Phase I and Phase II detoxification. Each of these phases requires specific nutrients to perform the work properly. In this program, the nutrients are supplied by the juices, raw soups, whole organic food, and supplements. They support the liver and enable it to break down the stuff we don't want and move it from one phase to the next. Without adequate nutrients, and especially antioxidants, detoxification can stall, which allows the free radicals that are formed during the intermediate process to proliferate, causing more damaged cells and further problems. But with plenty of nutrients, fat-soluble toxins that would otherwise be stored in fat cells and cell membranes can be converted into water-soluble forms that are subsequently excreted either through the kidneys, or via the bile that dumps into the colon.

In addition to detoxification, the liver performs numerous other tasks that are crucial to life and health. Many of these functions directly affect energy production, so when the liver is congested, its ability to produce energy is reduced. The main energy-producing functions include

- Regulating carbohydrate metabolism, which controls blood sugar
- Regulating protein metabolism, which produces proteins that transport substances such as fat and hormones
- Burning fat for fuel, as well as making cholesterol and fat and storing it
- Regulating hormonal metabolism, especially converting T4 to T3 (thyroid hormones); T4 goes mostly to the liver, where it is converted to T3

The liver holds a key to efficient metabolism, weight control, bowel health, and detoxification. Good function is especially crucial for weight loss, in that the liver is the major fat-burning organ in the body. Cleansing your liver can greatly improve your ablity to lose weight and increase your energy so you feel *more like exercising.*

When you regularly consume sweets and other processed carbohydrates (like bread, rolls, pizza, and pasta), junk food, artificial sweeteners, and beverages such as soda pop and alcohol, your liver converts most of these calories to fat, stores it, and you gain weight. Though not common, fat can build up in the liver, which can lead to "fatty liver." When this happens, something has gone wrong with the metabolism. It's known that fat accumulates in the liver with a number of conditions, the most common being obesity, and it is also associated with diabetes mellitus, high triglycerides, and heavy use of alcohol. For all these reasons, you want to get the bad carbs and junk out of your diet.

The liver stores toxins in its cells. The more toxins it stores, the more the liver functions are compromised. The liver can become congested just like the colon. When it is, excretion of bile is slowed down, and you'll be more prone to constipation. This leads to toxins lingering in the gut too long, and some will be absorbed back into the bloodstream. Toxins circulating in the system can cause water retention in certain areas of the body, especially the thighs, hips, and arms because the body holds on to the extra water to dilute toxins. This leads to cellulite — that unsightly, bumpy skin. A cleansed, well-functioning liver can greatly facilitate the loss of cellulite and water weight.

You may have a number of signs of liver congestion, even though all your liver-function blood tests appear normal. The tests used to determine liver function are not designed to show mild dysfunction, but rather liver damage. Because the liver is involved in so many critical functions, it can affect nearly every system in our body, including the nervous system, immune system, endocrine system, digestive system, and circulatory system. So if you have even a couple of the symptoms listed below, it's a great idea to get going on a liver cleanse

Symptoms of Liver Dysfunction

- Acne, allergies, or asthma
- Allergic conditions such as hay fever, hives, skin rashes, asthma
- Back pain
- Brown or dark spots on the skin, often called age spots or liver spots
- Bursitis
- Cancer
- Candidiasis
- Coated tongue or bad breath in the morning
- Fatigue, chronic fatigue syndrome
- Fluid retention, swollen legs, fingers, or toes
- Headaches: migraines, tension headaches, hormonal headaches, cluster headaches, pain in the eyes, vision problems
- High blood pressure
- Hypoglycemia, blood sugar instability
- Immune system weakness
- Inability to tolerate fatty foods
- Insomnia
- Irritable bowel syndrome (IBS)
- Kidney problems
- Lupus
- Mood changes, depression, "foggy" brain
- Nausea, abdominal pains, acid reflux
- Obesity
- Poor digestion, bloating, gas, weight gain, cellulite, and constipation
- Sinus problems
- Small bright red spots on the body (called cherry angiomas)
- Thin stools (diameter of a rope or pencil)

When you detoxify your liver, it should give a big sigh of relief and go on about its job of detoxifying, regulating metabolism, and burning fat. When the liver is working well, you'll feel and look better. Weight loss should be easy and natural, without excessive effort, and your immune system should function more efficiently, making it easier to stay healthy all year.

Gallbladder Detoxification

The liver and gallbladder are interconnected and work together. What affects one affects the other — both positively and negatively. One of the primary routes of eliminating toxins is through the bile, which is made in the liver and concentrated and stored in the gallbladder. Bile is needed to help break down fats and fat-soluble vitamins when it's secreted into the small intestine. Its other main function is to transport toxins from the liver. It's somewhat like a garbage truck, picking up toxic waste from the liver and transporting it down the bile duct "highway" into the bowels to be excreted through the colon.

Bile contains water, cholesterol, fat, bile salts, proteins, and bilirubin. If it contains too much cholesterol, bile salts, or bilirubin, due principally to inefficient liver function, it can sometimes harden into pieces of stonelike material called gallstones. There are two types of gallstones: cholesterol stones and pigment stones. Cholesterol stones are made from hardened cholesterol and are a yellow-green color. They account for about 80 percent of all gallstones. Pigment stones are made up principally of bilirubin, and are small, dark stones. The gallbladder can develop stones of all sizes, from hundreds of tiny ones to one large stone. If a stone gets stuck in the duct that carries bile from the liver to the small intestine, it can block the flow of bile, which causes inflammation and pain. In addition to forming stones from too much cholesterol (often related to a diet high in animal products) or too much bilirubin, they can form due to not enough bile salts, or because the gallbladder is not efficient enough to properly secrete bile.

Intense pain in the abdomen that radiates to the upper back can be an indication of gallstones. Ultrasound provides a definitive diagnosis. Approximately 20 percent of the women and 8 percent of the men over forty in the United States experience gallstones. Each year this leads to surgery to remove more than three hundred thousand gallbladders. It's far better to periodically complete a liver/gallbladder detox than to undergo the pain and expense of gallbladder surgery, which can adversely affect health thereafter. After all, your body was meant to have a gallbladder.

SYMPTOMS OF GALLBLADDER PROBLEMS

People can go for years with digestive problems and never realize that they may be related to the gallbladder because they're interrelated with other digestive symptoms. Constipation is one of the most commonly missed. The following list refers to symptoms associated with gallbladder problems, but bear in mind they could also be indicative of something else. But one thing is certain: it's better to cleanse and support your gallbladder at the first sign of problems than to lose it.

- Pain or tenderness under the rib cage on the right side
- Pain between shoulder blades
- Stools light or chalky colored
- Indigestion after eating, especially fatty or greasy foods
- Nausea
- Dizziness
- Bloating
- Gas
- Burping or belching
- Feeling of fullness or poor food digestion
- Diarrhea (or alternating from soft to watery stools)
- Constipation
- Headache over eyes, especially the right eye
- Bitter fluid reflux after eating
- Frequent need for laxatives

Diet for a Happy Liver and Gallbladder

There are certain foods, beverages, and lifestyle choices that can lead to health and wellness for the liver/gallbladder team. We call these "liver-friendly" foods and lifestyle choices. Those choices that undermine or interfere with this team's wellness are called "liver-unfriendly."

LIVER-FRIENDLY	LIVER-UNFRIENDLY
• Organic vegetables and vegetable juices	• Refined, processed, and canned foods
• Organic fruit	• Sweet foods, treats, desserts
• Raw nuts and seeds (organic)	• Fast foods (e.g. French fries, burgers, pizza, tacos)
• Legumes (organic)	• Deep-fried foods
• Whole grains (organic)	

(Continued)

LIVER-FRIENDLY	LIVER-UNFRIENDLY
• Free-range poultry and meats • Fish (wild caught) • Organic, free-range eggs • Good fats and oils (extra-virgin olive oil, coconut oil, fish oil) • Plenty of filtered or distilled water • Herb tea, green tea, or white tea • Exercise, especially aerobic • Positive, life-affirming attitudes, thoughts, and words • Moderate eating	• Refined flour products (bread, pasta, pizza dough, bagels) • Fatty meats, preserved meats, and cold cuts • Hydrogenated and partially hydrogenated fats (margarine) • Trans fats and polyunsaturated vegetable oils such as soy, corn, canola, sunflower, and safflower • Alcohol, coffee, soda pop • Sedentary lifestyle • Stress, anxiety, anger, worry, fear • Negative attitudes, thoughts, words • Overeating

The Five-Day Liver/Gallbladder Detox Program

A thorough detoxification program is best done at least twice a year, around the spring and the fall. For optimum health you may want to do a cleanse four times a year at each change of season.

An effective liver/gallbladder detoxification program includes these six important steps:

1. Reduce exposure to toxins — environmental and from processed, preserved foods.

2. Avoid coffee, alcohol, tobacco, junk food, all sweets, refined grains (wheat, rye, barley), soft drinks, and over-the-counter medications.

3. Eat a health-building, whole, organic foods diet — with plenty of raw vegetables, fruit, and fresh vegetable juices.

4. Exercise — sweat to eliminate toxins (saunas are also very helpful).

5. Drink plenty of water to flush toxins (2 to 2 ½ quarts).

6. Detoxify your liver and gallbladder using the programs below.

For five days, you will follow this menu plan and utilize juice and smoothie recipes in this book or your own favorites, as well as adding plenty of fresh raw vegetables and a small amount of low-sugar fruit. During this cleanse you will not be eating *any* animal products, but you can have as many fresh, raw vegetables, vegetable smoothies, and vegetable juices as you wish, so you should not experience hunger.

During the detoxification programs you will want to consume plenty of green vegetables in salads, juices, smoothies, raw soups, and lightly steamed vegetables. Choose from green leafy vegetables such as lettuce, spinach, Swiss chard, parsley, and mustard greens, as well as cruciferous vegetables such as broccoli, cauliflower, cabbage, Brussels sprouts, and kale. Greens are rich in essential vitamins, minerals, enzymes, phytonutrients, antioxidants, and chlorophyll. They help your body detoxify and reach an alkaline pH level, which is especially needed during a detox program.

You may want to supplement your diet with a concentrated, powdered greens formula that contains organically grown grasses such as wheatgrass, barley grass, oat grass, and other grasses. Many products also contain spirulina, sprouted grains, herbs, and green vegetables. The concentrated greens can help in the detoxification process (see Resources Guide).

Liver-Friendly Vegetables

Eat an abundance of the following liver-friendly vegetables during the five days of your detoxification program:

- Artichokes
- Beets
- Broccoli
- Brussels sprouts
- Cabbage
- Carrots
- Cauliflower
- Celery
- Chives
- Cucumber
- Eggplant
- Garlic
- Green beans
- Jerusalem artichokes (sun chokes)
- Kale
- Kohlrabi
- Lettuce
- Mustard greens
- Okra
- Onion
- Parsley
- Parsnips
- Peas
- Pumpkin
- Spinach
- Squash
- Sweet potatoes or yams

There are two menu plans that you may choose from. Both of these plans are very effective for cleansing the liver and gallbladder. Option 1 involves a little more preparation, but less expense. It's for people who have the time to prepare special juices and salads as outlined along with a few recommended herbs, but who do not want to spend much extra money on special liver/gallbladder cleansing herbs and teas. Option 2 is similar in many ways, but involves less time in preparation and entails purchasing cleansing herbs and teas. Choose from either option and follow as outlined for the full five days.

The best time to do this five-day program, if you work outside the home or go to school, is to start on the weekend, when you have a little more time to get personal things done. Then you can prepare the juices, smoothies, and salads ahead of time for the rest of the detox days and take what you need to work in a cooler for the remaining days. Option 2 is usually easier for people who work away from home, but you will still need to prepare mostly raw foods to take with you.

In addition to following the menu options, keep in mind the importance of a cleansed colon that moves freely. If you become constipated or your bowels are not moving every day, add fiber supplements and herbs (see chapter five on colon cleansing).

MENU PLAN FOR OPTION 1

Upon Rising

7:00 A.M. Or upon rising drink 1 cup filtered water
(distilled is best for detoxing)

7:15 A.M. Drink the Blended Citrus Shake

BLENDED CITRUS SHAKE

(you will consume this shake every morning)

*1 cup distilled or purified
    water*
*Juice of one lemon and
    one lime*
*1-inch piece of fresh
    gingerroot cut in pieces*
*1 to 5 cloves of garlic (day
    one use 1 garlic clove,
    day two use 2 garlic
    cloves, then continue
    adding one more garlic
    clover per day until day
    five when you'll end
    with 5 garlic cloves)*

*1 to 5 tablespoons of
    extra-virgin, cold-
    pressed olive oil (day
    one use 1 tablespoon,
    day two use 2
    tablespoons, continue
    adding one tablespoon
    per day until day five)*
*1 tablespoon virgin
    coconut oil (optional)**
*2 to 4 ice cubes (optional)
    (make ice cubes with
    filtered or distilled
    water)*

Place all ingredients into a blender and blend at high speed
for about one minute or until everything is well combined.
Pour into a large glass and drink it all. This shake will
stimulate your liver and begin to flush out toxins.

**A note about virgin coconut oil:* The liver likes to burn medium-chain fatty acids
that are contained in abundance in coconut oil. Read more about the wonderful
health- and weight-loss benefits of coconut oil in our book *The Coconut Diet.*

Breakfast

8:00 A.M.

- Beet-Cucumber Cleansing Cocktail (page 290). If desired, you can add the juice to a blender with an avocado; blend until smooth)
- 1 to 2 teaspoons Beet Salad (page 186). Beets are fabulous for liver detoxification and support, so you'll be consuming beet salad throughout the day
- Supplement: 1 to 2 capsules of the herb milk thistle or liver cleansing herbs (see Resources Guide)

10:00 A.M. Gallbladder Cleansing Cocktail (page 188)

10:30 A.M.

- 8 ounces of water with lemon (1/8 to 1/4 lemon)
- 1 to 2 teaspoons Beet Salad

11:30 A.M. Ginger or echinacea herbal tea, or use a commercial detox tea (see Resources Guide)

Lunch

12:00 Noon

- Choose any smoothie or raw soup recipe from the recipe section
- If you're still hungry, add a vegetable salad or raw vegetable sticks
- Supplement: 1 to 2 capsules of the herb milk thistle or liver-cleansing herbs

1:15 P.M. 1 to 2 teaspoons Beet Salad

3:00 P.M.

- Green Drink (page 187): Juice as many greens as you like. Start with a base of cucumber, celery, and lemon. To that add parsley, kale, spinach, sprouts, or any other greens. If juice is not possible, mix powdered greens in water
- 1 to 2 teaspoons Beet Salad

4:30 P.M.

- 8 ounces of water or herbal tea with lemon (1/8 to 1/4 lemon)
- 1 to 2 teaspoons Beet Salad

Dinner

6:00 P.M.*

- Carrot Salad with Lemon–Olive Oil Dressing (page 186)
- One cup Potassium-Rich Vegetable Broth (page 187)
- Vegetable salad or blended vegetable soup. You may substitute cooked artichokes, which are very liver supportive, but no dressing/dip other than olive oil and lemon juice
- Supplement: 1 to 2 capsules milk thistle or liver-cleansing herbs

*Avoid eating after 7:00 p.m. (except for Beet Salad) to give your liver and gallbladder a chance to do their work of detoxing while you sleep.

7:15 P.M. 1 to 2 teaspoons Beet Salad

8:30 P.M. Chamomile or peppermint herbal tea

MENU PLAN FOR OPTION 2

For recommendation of products that can work well with this program, see Resources Guide.

Upon Rising

7:00 A.M. Or upon rising drink 1 cup distilled or
    filtered water (distilled is best for detoxing)

7:15 A.M. Drink the Blended Citrus Shake

BLENDED CITRUS SHAKE

(you will consume this shake every morning)

1 to 2 cups distilled water
Juice of one lemon and
    one lime
1-inch piece of fresh
    gingerroot cut in pieces
1 to 5 cloves of garlic (day
    one use 1 garlic clove,
    day two use 2 garlic
    cloves, continue adding
    one garlic clove per
    day until day five when
    you will end with 5
    garlic cloves)

1 to 5 tablespoons of extra-
    virgin, cold-pressed
    olive oil (day one use
    1 tablespoon, day
    two use 2 tablespoons,
    continue adding one
    tablespoon per day
    until day five)
1 tablespoon virgin
    coconut oil (optional)*
2 to 4 ice cubes (optional)
    (make ice cubes with
    filtered or distilled water)

*A note about virgin coconut oil: The liver likes to burn medium-chain fatty acids that are contained in abundance in coconut oil. Read more about the wonderful health- and weight-loss benefits of coconut oil in our book *The Coconut Diet.*

Place all ingredients into a blender and blend at high speed for about one minute. Pour into a large glass and drink it all. This shake will stimulate your liver and begin to flush the toxins.

7:30 A.M. Drink two cups of detoxification tea and take liver/gallbladder herbal formulas as directed (see Resources Guide)

Breakfast

8:30 A.M.

- Beet-Cucumber Cleansing Cocktail (page 290). If desired, you can then add the juice to a blender with an avocado; blend until smooth) or
- Gallbladder Cleansing Cocktail (page 188) (alternate between these two choices)
- Optional: Add a concentrated greens powder to either choice (see Resources Guide)

Midmorning

- Drink two cups of detoxification tea
- Take liver/gallbladder herbal formulas as directed

Lunch

12:00 Noon

- **On Days 1 and 5:** You may have a vegetable salad, raw vegetable sticks, or lightly steamed vegetables like broccoli or cooked artichoke. Or choose from any of the juice, smoothie, or raw soup recipes. For salad dressing choose from olive oil, lemon juice, avocado, garlic, Bragg Liquid Aminos, or any spices or herbs

- **On Days 2 through 4:** Choose any juice, smoothie, or raw soup recipe from the recipe section. You will not be consuming any solid food on these days

Midafternoon

- Drink two cups of detoxification tea
- Take liver/gallbladder herbal formulas as directed

Dinner

6:00 P.M.*

- **On Days 1 and 5:** You may have a vegetable salad, raw vegetable sticks, or lightly steamed vegetables like broccoli or cooked artichoke. Or choose from any of the juice, smoothie, or raw soup recipes. For salad dressing choose from olive oil, lemon juice, avocado, garlic, Bragg Liquid Aminos, or any spices or herbs

---

*Avoid eating after 7:00 p.m. to give your liver and gallbladder a chance to do their work of detoxing while you sleep.

- **On Days 2 through 4:** Choose any juice, smoothie, or raw soup recipe from the recipe section, or have one cup Potassium-Rich Vegetable Broth (page 187). You will not be consuming any solid food on these days

Evening: Herb teas of your choice

Summary of Liver/Gallbladder Detox Programs

- Increase consumption of water, vegetable juice, and herb teas to flush toxins.
- Follow Detoxification menu plan, either Option 1 or Option 2.
- Drink Blended Citrus Shake every morning.
- Eat liver-friendly foods and eliminate liver-unfriendly foods (see box page 171).
- Eat no animal foods during this cleanse.
- Take herbal liver cleanse formulas and detoxing teas (use according to product directions) if following Option 2.
- Add aerobic exercises to increase heart rate and cause sweating.
- Take saunas or hot baths during the cleanse to facilitate sweating.

When you have finished your liver/gallbladder cleanse, eat only whole foods and follow the basic cleansing steps until you are ready to go on to either the Kidney Flush or a second liver/gallbladder cleanse that includes an optional sixth day of intensive gallbladder cleansing (see below).

Why Complete an Intensive Gallbladder Flush?

You may be one of millions of people who have one or many gallstones that have accumulated in the gallbladder or liver. These stones can be in the form of little rocks, sand, or "muddy substances." If you suspect you have gallstones, or are over forty and have eaten a typical American diet, or have never done a liver or gallbladder cleanse and just want to be sure your gallbladder is as clean as possible, you may want to try the Intensive Gallbladder Flush.

Before you do this flush, you will need to complete at least two of the five-day liver/gallbladder detoxification programs as outlined above. These programs will help to soften stones and increase bile solubility. The Intensive Gallbladder Flush will aggressively go after stubborn stones that may still be in your gallbladder or liver. If you wish, you can take a break for a week or two before starting your second cleanse, but during that break avoid animal products as much as possible and eat a low-fat diet, except for good fats that include fish oil, virgin coconut oil, and extra-virgin olive oil.

On your second five-day liver/gallbladder detox, plan to add an extra day, such as a Saturday when you have some time to devote to yourself. On the sixth day, follow the Intensive Gallbladder Flush exactly as outlined below. On the seventh day you may pass stones of various colors.

NOTE: If you should try the Intensive Gallbladder Flush prematurely, the gallbladder could release a large stone that could block the bile duct, which would require immediate surgery. Before embarking on the Intensive Sixth-Day Gallbladder Flush, you may wish to consult your health care professional.

If you have problems with constipation or a sluggish colon, you could benefit by using the Colon Cleansing fiber formulas (see page 151) during your second liver/ gallbladder detoxification program. You may want to take an enema as outlined in chapter five on page 157 to be sure your colon is moving efficiently before you begin the Intensive Sixth-Day Gallbladder Flush. And make sure you eat no animal products during this flush.

The Intensive Sixth-Day Gallbladder Flush

NOTE: Only do this after you have completed two previous Five-Day Liver/Gallbladder Detox programs. The Intensive Gallbladder Flush is done on the sixth day of your second Liver/Gallbladder Detox Program. I no longer recommend using Epsom salts since it is hard on your organs of elimination.

Choose a day like Saturday for the Intensive Flush, when you can rest most of the day.

- Take no medications (except prescription medication that is mandatory) or nutritional supplements on this day.
- Drink only fresh vegetable juices for breakfast and lunch.
- Eat no solid food on this day.
- After 2:00 p.m. do not drink juices, but drink plenty of water to which you can add lemon.

- **9:45 p.m.** Pour 1/2 cup of extra-virgin olive oil into a saucepan and add 1/2 cup of apple juice or grapefruit juice, gently warmed. Pour the mixture in a jar and shake or pour in a blender and process. Mix thoroughly and drink it all down within five minutes. You may want to rinse your mouth after this.

- **10:00 p.m.** (or sooner) Lie down in bed on your right side immediately after drinking this mixture. Try to lie still for at least twenty minutes; hopefully, you can go to sleep.

- The next morning, upon awakening, drink one cup of hot water with lemon.

- One hour after, you may have fresh vegetable juice.

- You may have a fresh garden salad for lunch or a vegetable smoothie or raw soup.

WHAT SHOULD I EXPECT?

Though this program does not offer an appealing taste, it's worth it because it works. Here's what you can expect.

You may experience diarrhea. Sometime during the morning of the seventh day, you should pass gallstones, sand, or mud. Gallstones are usually green and pea-sized, but can range in size from that of lemon seeds to dimes, and they float. Sand or mud looks about like it sounds. Colors of stones can range from tan, black, and light to dark green to turquoise. I only mention this so you won't be too alarmed by what you see. The upside of what to expect is greatly improved digestion.

LIVER AND GALLBLADDER DETOX RECIPES AND PRODUCTS

BEET SALAD

2 tablespoons extra-virgin, cold-pressed olive oil

Juice of 1/2 lemon

1 cup raw beets, finely grated or very finely chopped (or use the pulp from your juicer after making beet juice)

Whisk the olive oil and lemon juice together and mix with the beets.

Dash of cinnamon (optional)

Eat one to two teaspoons of this salad every two to three hours during the day for five days. You may get tired of eating beets all day, but remember how great it is for your liver. Eating a few teaspoons of this salad every couple hours is a small price to pay to help your precious liver. Don't be alarmed if your stools or urine are red from the beets.

CARROT SALAD WITH LEMON–OLIVE OIL DRESSING

1 cup shredded carrots (or carrot pulp)

1 tablespoon extra-virgin, cold-pressed olive oil

1 tablespoon lemon juice

Dash of cinnamon (optional)

Place finely shredded carrots, or carrot pulp leftover from juicing, in a bowl. If shredding the carrots, they should be a mushy consistency; use a food processor or fine grater.

(It's easiest to use carrot pulp.) For the dressing, combine extra-virgin, cold-pressed olive oil with fresh lemon juice and a dash of cinnamon (optional). Whisk together. You may add more dressing, but not less. Pour the dressing over the shredded carrots (or carrot pulp) and mix well.

GREEN DRINK

Preferably in the afternoon, drink 10 ounces freshly juiced green vegetables — cucumber, parsley, spinach, kale, celery, or any other green herb or vegetable. Add fresh lemon juice and/or freshly juiced gingerroot to pep up the flavor. Fresh mint also makes a nice addition with cucumber and other milder-tasting greens.

POTASSIUM-RICH VEGETABLE BROTH

This vegetable broth provides important nutrients, especially minerals, your body needs during the cleansing process. Eat one to two cups of broth daily.

2 to 3 cups chopped fresh green beans (string beans) (frozen is acceptable when fresh is unavailable)	Purified water, for steaming
	1 to 3 tablespoons chopped parsley
2 to 3 cups chopped zucchini	1 tablespoon chopped garlic
2 to 3 stalks celery	Seasonings and herbs, to taste
	Coconut oil (optional)

Steam the green beans, zucchini, and celery over purified water until soft, but still green and not mushy. Place the cooked vegetables, plus the raw parsley and garlic, in a blender and puree until smooth. Add a bit of the steaming water, as needed, but keep the broth fairly thick. Season to taste with minced ginger, cayenne, vegetable seasoning, or herbs of your choice. Add coconut oil, if desired.

MAKES ABOUT 6 SERVINGS

GALLBLADDER CLEANSING COCKTAIL

1 handful parsley
4 medium carrots,
scrubbed well, green
tops removed, ends
trimmed

2 stalks celery with leaves,
washed, ends trimmed
1/2 lemon, peeled

Bunch up the parsley and push it through the juicer feed tube with the carrots, celery, and lemon. Stir the juice and pour into a glass. If you want a more substantial drink, you can pour the juice into a blender, then add an avocado. Blend and serve in a glass or bowl, or you can make it thick like a soup and eat with a spoon by adding more avocado and less of the juice. Drink as soon as possible to maximize the nutritional value, or store in the refrigerator, covered, or take in a thermos.

RECOMMENDATIONS FOR ADDITIONAL FRESH VEGETABLE JUICE

- Carrot, beet, and cucumber juice
- Carrot, celery, and endive or kale juice
- Carrot, beet, and coconut milk
- Carrot and spinach

NOTE: If you are sugar sensitive (hypoglycemic or diabetic) and react to carrots or beets, then use cucumber and more greens, and flavor with lemon juice and ginger. You can also add avocado to the juice and blend until smooth.

Milk Thistle (Silymarin)

Take one or two capsules of the herb milk thistle with each meal. Milk thistle contains potent liver-cleansing compounds. Silymarin, the most active ingredient in milk thistle, enhances liver function. It also has excellent antioxidant properties that help prevent damage to the liver. Or you can use a liver-cleansing herbal combination that contains milk thistle.

Liver/Gallbladder Cleansing Herbs

There are various cleansing herbal formulas for detoxifying the liver and gallbladder, improving liver function, increasing bile flow, reducing swelling, and purifying the blood. They can be partnered with herbs used to strengthen the liver's glandular and organ functions. Such herbs help remove fat deposits associated with consuming too many unhealthy foods, damaged fats, sugar, and alcohol, as well as chemical exposure. For more information, see Resources Guide.

Liver/Gallbladder Cleansing, Stimulating, and Protecting Herbs:

It's not recommended that you formulate your own combinations of these herbs, since they are not combined in equal amounts, but rather look for liver/gallbladder cleansing products that contain some or all of these (see Resources Guide).

- Artichoke leaf
- Barberry root bark
- Black walnut hull
- Burdock root
- Cardamom seed
- Cinnamon bark
- Clove
- Curcumin
- Dandelion root
- Fennel seed
- Garlic
- Gentian root
- Gingerroot
- Goldenseal root
- Horsetail herb
- Juniper berry
- Licorice root
- Mandrake root
- Milk thistle
- Oregon grape root
- Parsley root
- Pau d'Arco bark
- Schizandra
- Turmeric
- Uva ursi leaf
- Wormwood
- Yellow dock root

Lipotropic Formula (Great for the Gallbladder)

A lipotropic formula includes choline, methionine, taurine, HCL betaine, folic acid, and vitamin B6. This combination of nutrients helps remove fat from the liver and increases bile solubility. Take as directed (see Resources Guide).

The Liver and Emotions

The liver is a doorway into our emotional library. Unexpressed or denied emotions have the ability to shut down important liver functions. Watch for emotions that surface when working on the liver; anger is a typical emotion to pop up. More than any other organ, the liver is affected by negative thoughts and feelings. Anger, hate, rage, fear, jealousy, resentment, depression, self-pity, self-unforgiveness, self-rejection, self-bitterness, and hopelessness have a powerfully detrimental impact on the liver.

Kidney Cleansing

When we cleanse, it's important to include the kidneys, as they are one of the five primary organs for eliminating toxins from the body. The kidneys filter the blood, returning most of the water and many of the dissolved substances back into the bloodstream. What's left is called the urine, which passes through the ureters to the bladder for storage, and finally through the urethra for elimination. Toxins and metabolic waste are eliminated through the urine.

The kidneys have many other important functions, such as the regulation of blood volume and blood pressure, the regulation of ion levels in the blood, and regulation of the pH of the blood, so it's crucial that they function at peak efficiency.

During cleansing, the kidneys must process more toxic substances than normal, including proteins, salts, and chemicals. If they are congested, we can experience mild symptoms such as water retention or more severe symptoms such as inflammation of kidney tissue. Concentrated protein wastes can cause inflammation of kidney filtering tissues (nephritis) causing the bloodstream to become overloaded with toxins. It's also well known that the emotions of fear and insecurity can cause kidney imbalances.

A number of herbs are beneficial in strengthening and toning the kidneys. They help increase urine flow, reduce inflammation, and remove uric acid and other crystalline formations. The Five-Day Kidney Flush that follows contains natural foods and herbs that support and cleanse the kidneys.

The Five-Day Kidney Flush

- **Throughout the day:** Drink a minimum of ten 8-ounce glasses (2 1/2 quarts) of distilled or purified water (distilled is best) throughout the day. The kidneys need water to cleanse efficiently, so drink, drink, drink your water!

Upon Rising

- Drink 1 cup of herbal tea such as agrimony, marshmallow, juniper, or buchu. (These can be found at health food stores.) These diuretic herbs will help rid the body of excess water and they benefit the urinary tract as well
- Drink fresh juice such as Kidney Tonic (page 195) or Cranberry Water (page 195)

Breakfast

8:00 A.M.

- Awesome Green Smoothie (page 196) or
- One of the vegetable juice recipes (pages 290 to 301)
- Optional: Add a concentrated greens powder to either choice (see Resources Guide)

Midmorning

- Nettle tea (and kidney herbal supplement, as desired — see Resources Guide)
- Cranberry Water

Lunch

12:00 Noon

- **On Days 1 and 5:** You may have a vegetable salad, raw vegetable sticks, or lightly steamed vegetables like broccoli or cooked artichoke. Or choose from any of the juice, smoothie, or raw soup recipes. For salad dressing choose from olive oil, lemon juice, avocado, garlic, and any spices or herbs

- **On Days 2 through 4:** Choose any juice, smoothie, or raw soup recipes from the recipe section. You will not be consuming any solid food on these days

Midafternoon

- Cranberry Water (and kidney herbal supplement, as desired)

Dinner

6:00 P.M.*

- **On Days 1 and 5:** You may have a vegetable salad, raw vegetable sticks, or lightly steamed vegetables like broccoli or cooked artichoke. Or choose from any of the juice, smoothie, or raw soup recipes. For salad dressing choose from olive oil, lemon juice, avocado, garlic, or any spices or herbs
- **On Days 2 through 4:** Choose any juice, smoothie, or raw soup recipes from the recipe section, or have one cup Potassium-Rich Vegetable Broth (page 187). You will not be consuming any solid food on these days

*Avoid eating after 7:00 p.m. to give your kidneys a chance to do their work of detoxing while you sleep.

Evening: Herbal tea (and herbal supplement, as desired)

KIDNEY-CLEANSING RECIPES AND PRODUCTS

CRANBERRY WATER

Mix 1 to 2 teaspoons unsweetened cranberry concentrate in 8 to 10 ounces water. (Unsweetened cranberry concentrate can be purchased at health food stores.) Add a little stevia, if desired. (Do not use any artificial sweeteners, including Splenda.)

NETTLE TEA

The herb nettles is used traditionally for kidney cleansing and support; it helps eliminate uric acid. Drink 1 cup of this tea each day.

KIDNEY TONIC

1 cucumber, peeled if not organic
1 handful parsley
1 stalk celery

1/4 lemon, peeled, or a handful of mint
1/2-inch piece gingerroot

Cut the cucumber in half and juice. Bunch up the parsley and juice followed by the celery, lemon, mint, and ginger. (Parsley and celery are kidney tonic juices.)

NOTE: Cucumber, watermelon, cantaloupe with seeds, asparagus, lemon, kiwifruit, and parsley are all considered natural diuretics.

AWESOME GREEN SMOOTHIE

1 small to medium cucumber, peeled if not organic
2 cups spinach, washed
1 small to medium avocado, peeled with pit removed

1 tablespoon virgin coconut oil (optional)
Juice from one lime or lemon
Pinch of stevia to sweeten (optional)

Cut the cucumber into chunks, and add to the blender and blend well. Add spinach and blend. Cut the avocado into chunks and add to blender along with coconut oil (if using) and other ingredients. Blend until smooth and then pour into glasses or bowls.

SERVES 2 (YOU CAN STORE THE SECOND SERVING IN A JAR FOR USE LATER IN THE DAY)

KIDNEY CLEANSING HERBAL SUPPLEMENTS

You may also wish to take an herbal supplement that will detoxify the kidneys. It is not recommended that you formulate your own combinations of these herbs, since they are not combined in equal amounts (see Resources Guide). Look for the following herbs that are cleansing to the kidneys, bladder, and the entire urinary system:

- Agrimony
- Buchu
- Burdock root
- Gingerroot
- Gravel root
- Hydrangea root
- Juniper berries
- Lobelia leaf
- Marshmallow root
- Nettles
- Parsley leaf
- Uva ursi

Summary of Kidney-Detox Program

- Increase consumption of water, vegetable juice, and herb tea to flush toxins.
- Follow kidney detoxification menu plan.
- Take herbal formulas and detoxing teas (use according to product directions).

CHAPTER SEVEN

More Detox Programs

Now that you have successfully completed your colon, liver, gallbladder, and kidney cleansing programs, you can move on to some special cleanses that will help address specific problems. The Lung Cleanse, Skin Cleanse, and Lymphatic Cleanse can be carried out at the same time as any of the other cleanses as a means of augmenting and facilitating the removal of toxins. The Candida, parasite, and heavy-metal detox programs have specific protocols that must be followed carefully for optimum results.

For all the programs, follow Steps 1 through 5 throughout the process.

- **STEP 1**: Eat only whole, alkalizing, organic, non-GMO foods, and make 50 to 75 percent of the foods raw.

- **STEP 2**: Remove as many sources of toxicity as possible.
- **STEP 3**: Drink plenty of purified water (2 to 2 1/2 quarts).
- **STEP 4**: Add fresh vegetable juices to your diet at least once or twice a day.
- **STEP 5**: Complete periodic juice fasts for one to three days (except during a heavy-metal detox).

The Lung Cleanse

The lungs are one of the five major organs of elimination. The lungs breathe in air that principally contains oxygen, nitrogen, hydrogen, and carbon, then processes it by extracting what the body needs to produce fuel from the foods we eat. The lungs then expel carbon dioxide gas, along with some of the toxic wastes that have been produced in the body. It is crucial throughout the cleansing process to keep the lungs functioning at peak efficiency. Use the following breathing exercises to assist your lungs in their capacity as organs of elimination.

DEEP CLEANSING BREATHS

Breathe deeply from your diaphragm by filling up your belly and upper chest (let your belly stick out as you breathe in); hold for a count of two, and then expel the air. This exercise can be done throughout the day; do a minimum of six times. Try to be conscious of your breathing, especially if you are anxious or under pressure, so you don't hold your breath.

AEROBIC EXERCISE PROMOTES DEEP BREATHING

"Aerobic" means in the presence of oxygen. Add a program of aerobic exercise to your daily routine for lifelong health and wellness—the lungs and the entire body will benefit. Great aerobic exercises that promote deep breathing include brisk walking, snow shoeing, jogging, bicycling, hiking, aerobic dance, step aerobics classes, swimming, or rebounding. Find something you enjoy and have the energy to perform, and try to exercise outside as often as possible, as outdoor air is usually less polluted than indoor air. A walk or jog in the fresh air is also nourishing to your spirit.

RELEASE EMOTIONS LIKE SADNESS AND GRIEF

Negative emotions, particularly sadness and grief, are known to inhibit or impede lung health. Holding on to grief, sadness, and sorrow often will lead to shallow breathing and lung contraction. These repressed emotions become toxic, as they interfere with the delivery of nutrients and the removal of waste products through the lungs. (See chapter eight for more information on emotional cleansing.)

The Skin Cleanse

The skin covers the entire surface area of the body, making it the largest organ of elimination. The skin has many important functions, including the regulation of body temperature and the elimination of toxins through sweating. It aids all the other channels of elimination during the detoxification process, so it is vitally important that the skin pores do not get clogged. There are a number of ways to facilitate and support the skin so it can function optimally in the cleansing process.

DRY SKIN BRUSHING

The outer layer of the skin, known as the epidermis, can become clogged with dead skin cells, thus inhibiting the natural elimination of toxic waste through the pores. Brushing the skin with a natural bristle or vegetable fiber brush facilitates elimination of this waste from the skin. Brushing the skin when dry helps to open the pores, increase circulation, stimulate the lymphatic system, and eliminate dead skin cells. Cleansing your skin on a regular basis will reduce stress on the liver and kidneys because there will be less toxic load on them if the pores are kept open.

You can purchase a natural vegetable fiber brush at your health food store. Do not use a synthetic brush, as it scratches the skin. Brush the skin every day when dry, before bathing or showering. This type of brushing is best done in the morning as it can be too stimulating and can interrupt sleep if done before bedtime.

- Start with the bottoms of your feet, and then continue brushing up the legs using circular motions. Always stroke toward the heart, gently but firmly.
- Use circular, counterclockwise strokes on the abdomen.
- Always move outward to inward, starting with the hands and moving up the arms.
- Brush lightly around the breasts; do not brush the nipples.
- Brush the entire body for best results.
- Place sea salt on the brush to cause the pores to open more.
- Wash your brush every few weeks and let it dry.

CONVENTIONAL AND INFRARED SAUNAS

Sweating is the body's natural means for regulating body heat. A sauna induces perspiration for therapeutic purposes, which causes toxins to be released through sweat. Sweat is produced from lymphatic fluid, and heat causes toxins to be released from the cells into the lymph. This process lightens the toxic load on the liver and kidneys by providing an additional channel of elimination of wastes that are released during the cleansing process.

Conventional saunas heat the air to fairly high temperatures, usually between 180 and 235 degrees Fahrenheit. These high temperatures increase the heart rate, and can put a strain on the heart of sensitive individuals. If it's difficult for you to stay in a conventional sauna, one alternative is the infrared sauna. Infrared heat is a form of radiant heat. This type of sauna heats only 20 percent of the air itself, whereas 80 percent directly heats objects like your body. Infrared heat can be used at lower temperatures (110 to 130 degrees), which enables it to penetrate more deeply and induce sweating without draining your energy or putting an undo strain on your body. Infrared saunas allow your body to secrete up to three times more perspiration than conventional saunas.

Infrared saunas have been shown to facilitate the removal of environmental toxins such as PCBs, pesticide residues, plastic toxins, as well as heavy metals that are difficult to remove by conventional cleansing programs. The effects of a sauna can be invigorating and energizing as your body's toxic load is lightened.

THERAPEUTIC BATHS

If you don't have access to a sauna, you can create a therapeutic bath at home to help your body sweat. The hot bath brings toxins to the surface of the skin and opens pores so they can be eliminated.

- Fill a tub with water that is as hot as you can comfortably tolerate, preferably filtered water (water filters for tubs and showers or the whole house are now widely available).
- Plan to stay in the tub for about ten to twenty minutes for maximum benefit.
- Add therapeutic ingredients
  - Epsom salts contain magnesium, which helps muscles relax, and sulfur, which aids in detoxification; 1 cup is a good start.
  - Ginger is a favorite of mine. You can juice fresh gingerroot and pour 1/8 to 1/4 cup ginger juice into the water. Ginger helps the body sweat and draws out toxins.
  - Baking soda and sea salt make a good alkalinizing bath; add 1 cup baking soda and 1 cup sea salt to hot water.

EXERCISE

Aerobic exercise such as walking, jogging, swimming, bicycling, racquet sports, snow shoeing, step aerobics classes, dancing, and rebounding increase your circulation and induce perspiration, thus promoting excretion of toxins more efficiently through the skin. You can combine aerobic exercises with strength training like weight lifting. Increase the time and intensity of your workout so you sweat as much as possible. Shower immediately after a workout to remove the toxins so they will not be reabsorbed.

WATER

Drink the recommended eight to ten glasses of purified, distilled, or alkaline water throughout the day. It is vitally important to get enough water during the detox programs in order to flush toxins from your body, but it's even more crucial when you are perspiring and losing fluids. Drink an additional one to two glasses of water for every hour you are sweating, either from saunas, baths, or vigorous exercise.

Lymphatic System Cleanse

The lymphatic system is one of the supporting channels of elimination that is responsible for getting rid of toxins. However, since the lymphatic system does not have an active pump, it's dependent primarily on exercise and breathing to move the lymph through its many vessels. Breathing acts like a pressure pump to move lymph, and exercise pushes against the lymphatic vessels and squeezes them, thereby pushing the lymph along in a type of "milking action."

The lymphatic vessels function as the garbage collection system. They pick up the by-products of cellular respiration that have been excreted into the intracellular fluid and carry them through the body for elimination. Therefore, keeping the lymph moving freely through the vessels is a vitally important step in the detoxification process.

SKIN CLEANSING FACILITATES LYMPHATIC CLEANSING

Dry brushing, saunas, therapeutic baths, exercise, and drinking plenty of water all contribute to cleansing the lymphatic system. In addition, add the following cleansing steps:

DEEP BREATHING

Deep breathing changes the pressure differential from the abdomen to the chest and is one of the two ways that lymph is moved through the vessels. Use your diaphragm to fill up the belly and upper chest with air, hold for a count of two, and expel the air. Do this several times a day. Remember to breathe deeply throughout the day, and be sure not to hold your breath when you're tense.

LYMPHASIZER (HEALTHY SWINGER)

The lymphasizer, also known as the healthy swinger, is an excellent aid to your lymphatic detoxification because it will actively move the lymph and blood through the body when you lie down on it. Dr. Shizuo Inoue developed this machine after observing the rhythmic, side-to-side movement of healthy, well-toned fish. This type of machine creates a wavelike motion up and down the spine as it gently massages the body and oxygenates muscles, tissues, and cells. It moves lymph through the lymphatic vessels so it can efficiently deliver its load of toxins to the organs of elimination.

It's very beneficial for those with circulation problems, those with diabetes, or those using steroids. With this machine, you can have a low-impact workout that requires no active movement. You can lie on the floor with your feet in the grooves and get the aerobic benefits for your lymphatic system equal to a half hour of exercise in about ten to fifteen minutes.

The lymphasizer provides a simple exercise without applying any stress on the spine or other body parts. Simply lie down and the machine will move your body from side to side. This simple side-to-side motion maintains a proper energy balance and oxygen supply to the body. Regular use of this relaxing massage movement stimulates your body and achieves relaxation and stress reduction. A sense of well-being arises from the massaging, swing action that is immediately noticeable.

Though this machine is a great addition for everyone, it can be excellent for the disabled, for anyone with hip, knee, or ankle problems, and those who for other medical reasons are unable to even bounce slowly on a rebounder (see Resources Guide).

LYMPHATIC MASSAGE

Lymphatic drainage massage can be quite helpful in promoting lymphatic system detoxification. The massage therapist works on the muscles of the body that push against the walls of the main lymphatic system vessels, thus aiding in the movement of the lymph that carries toxins to the channels of elimination.

The Candida Detoxification Program

Candida albicans are usually benign yeasts (or fungus) that naturally inhabit the folds and creases of the digestive tract and the vaginal tract in women. They normally live in harmonious relationship with beneficial intestinal flora, also known as "probiotics." In healthy people, *Candida albicans* does not present a problem because it is kept in check by friendly bacteria that also inhabit the gut.

These good bacteria, however, can be easily destroyed by the use of antibiotics and other medications, allowing *Candida albicans* to flourish. Other factors connected with our twenty-first-century lifestyle such as diets rich in sugar, refined carbohydrates, and alcohol, along with the use of birth control pills (pregnancy, hormonal changes), and stress encourage yeasts to grow.

Thought to affect more than forty million Americans, *Candida albicans* is now being recognized as a complex medical syndrome known as "chronic candidiasis" or "yeast syndrome." These organisms attach themselves to the intestinal wall, where they compete with cells and ultimately the entire body for nutrients, thus creating nutrient deficiencies. This overgrowth of yeast is believed to cause widespread symptoms in virtually every system of the body, with the gastrointestinal, genitourinary, endocrine, nervous, and immune systems being the most susceptible.

SYMPTOMS OF CANDIDIASIS

- Canker sores
- Chemical sensitivities
- Depression
- Digestive problems
- Ear and sinus irritation
- Fatigue
- Feeling "sick all over"
- Immune system dysfunction
- Intense itching
- Ringworm
- Vaginitis
- Weight gain

If you think you may have a yeast overgrowth, take the Candida Questionnaire on page 216.

PREDISPOSING FACTORS

Chronic candidiasis has many predisposing factors, such as altered bowel flora, decreased digestive secretions, dietary factors such as consuming too much sugar and too many other high-carbohydrate foods, drugs (particularly antibiotics), immune dysfunction, impaired liver function, nutrient deficiencies, and underlying disease states. To simply go after the yeasts and kill them off, whether using natural or synthetic antifungal agents, will not get to the root cause of why you developed candidiasis in the first place. It's a lot like cutting leaves off a weed. It's vitally important to address all the factors that predisposed you to yeast overgrowth and get to the root of the problem so it doesn't return in the future.

CORRECTING THE PROBLEM

In addition to using antifungal agents, it's very important to address the predisposing factors. Here's what I recommend.

Follow a Candida-Control Diet

Incorporate a healthy, low-carb diet, such as the one in *The Coconut Diet*, which has over seventy recipes, during a candida detox program. I recommend virgin coconut oil because it contains fatty acids that help kill yeasts. The early phases of the diet eliminate grains, fruit, alcohol, sugars, and other carbs that quickly turn to sugar such as refined flour and starches, which *Candida albicans* is known to feed on. All natural sugars should also be eliminated when cleansing the body of yeasts. Sugars are a primary food for yeasts. Milk and dairy products need to be omitted because milk lactose promotes over-growth of yeasts. And all mold- and yeast-containing foods such as alcohol, cheese, dried fruit, bread, and pea-nuts must be completely avoided. Food allergens should also be eliminated. Candidiasis sufferers may need to avoid these foods for a number of months, as *Candida albicans* infection*s* are known to be opportunistic and very difficult to overcome if the condition is systemic (meaning that the yeast has spread to other areas out-side the digestive tract). It's best to stick with this diet until you are symptom free and yeast free, which can be determined by a stool test. (See box on page 224, Foods to Avoid During a Parasite [or Candida] Cleanse.)

Include Plenty of Virgin Coconut Oil in Your Diet

Research shows that the medium-chain fatty acids in coco-nut oil kill *Candida albicans*. Caprylic acid is one of the fatty acids it contains that has been used successfully to fight candida. William Crook, MD, the author of *The Yeast Connection* and developer of the Candida Questionnaire, reports that many physicians have used caprylic acid successfully for yeast overgrowth and that it works espe-cially well for those patients who have adverse reactions to antifungal drugs. Coconut oil also contains two other medium-chain fatty acids, lauric and capric acid, that have been shown to kill *C. albicans*. A study done at the Univer-sity of Iceland showed "capric acid, a 10-carbon saturated fatty acid, causes the fastest and most effective killing of all three strains of *Candida albicans* tested, leaving the cytoplasm disorganized and shrunken because of a disrupted or disintegrated plasma membrane. Lauric acid, a 12-carbon saturated fatty acid, was the most active at lower concentrations and after a longer incubation time." This study makes the case that all the medium-chain fatty acids in coconut oil work together to help you get rid of *Candida albicans.* (To order larger quantities of virgin coconut oil for a significant savings, see the Resources Guide.)

Assist Digestive Secretions
A major step in treating candidiasis is improving digestive secretions. Gastric hydrochloric acid, pancreatic enzymes, and bile all inhibit the overgrowth of yeasts and prevent its penetration into the surfaces of the small intestine. Decreased secretion of any of these components can lead to a proliferation of *Candida albicans.* And modern society offers numerous factors that decrease HCL; stress, food excesses, especially over-consuming fats and proteins, and chemical use, along with aging (over fifty) can reduce HCL. Harmful emotions such as fear, worry, and anxiety also decrease gastric secretions. Other conditions associated with low stomach acid include malabsorption, pernicious anemia, rosacea, eczema, anemia, food allergies, thyroid dysfunction, vitiligo, atrophic gastritis, Helicobacter pylori infection of the stomach, and gastric

cancer. You can take the gastric challenge test to measure the amount of stomach acid you have. Most holistic doctors have the materials to perform this test.

Supplementation with hydrochloric acid (HCL betaine), pepsin, pancreatic enzymes, and nutrients that improve bile flow are all helpful in treating chronic candidiasis. The *proteases* (pancreatic enzymes) are enzymes that break down proteins and are mostly responsible for keeping the small intestines free of parasites (yeasts, bacteria, protozoa, and worms). (A deficiency in pancreatic enzymes is also one of the reasons some people experience excessive hair breakage, slow growth or loss of hair, or poor fingernail growth.) Supplementation should include HCL betaine, pancreatic enzymes, and a lipotropic formula to promote bile flow (the formula should include choline, methionine, and/or cysteine). (See the Resources Guide for recommendations.)

Support the Immune System
A compromised immune system leads to yeast overgrowth, and *Candida albicans* infection promotes damage to the immune system. It's a vicious circle. Tests can document immune dysfunction, but they are expensive. A practical (and free) evaluation is to look at your health history. A history of viral infections including colds and flu, sinus infections, outbreaks of cold sores or genital herpes, prostatitis in men, and vaginal infections in women are indicative of immune dysfunction.

Supplementation with antioxidants, which include vitamins C and E, beta-carotene, selenium, and glutathione (found in abundance in vegetables and especially their juices), along with virgin coconut oil (to control candida) can be very helpful in improving immune function.

Detoxify the Liver

Drs. Michael Murray and Joseph Pizzorno, authors of *The Encyclopedia of Natural Medicine*, say that improving liver health and promoting detoxification may be critical factors in the successful treatment of candidiasis. They note that damage to the liver is often an underlying factor in chronic candidiasis as well as in chronic fatigue. Studies with mice have shown that even slight liver damage causes *Candida albicans* to run rampant.

Chapter six outlines the liver-detox program. It's best to complete a liver/gallbladder detoxification before embarking on the candida detoxification program.

Take Probiotics

Probiotics, which are strains of beneficial intestinal flora such as *Lactobacillus acidophilus* and *Bactobacillus bifidum*, promote a healthy intestinal environment. It's very important that as you kill off the yeast, you replace the good bacteria. Choose a good probiotic supplement as part of your wellness plan.

Take an Antifungal Compound

In addition to coconut oil, you may benefit from taking a yeast-killing agent such as an herbal supplement that contains the herbs oregano and olive leaf or a product with cellulase and protease (doesn't cause die-off symptoms as the other products do).

Drink Plenty of Water

It is very important to drink plenty of purified water to flush your system as you kill off yeasts — aim for one quart of water for every fifty pounds of weight. It will help to reduce die-off symptoms (discomfort as the yeast in your system dies) and will promote weight loss and good hydration.

THE HERXHEIMER REACTION AND CANDIDIASIS

Be aware that as yeasts die, your symptoms may worsen for a short time or you may experience some reactions such as headaches or diarrhea. Such reactions are known as the Herxheimer Reaction (die-off effect), which is the result of the rapid killing of microorganisms and absorption of large quantities of yeast toxins, cell particles, and antigens. Hang in there. Your health will improve if you stick with the program. You'll be delighted with how you feel when you finally rid yourself of this obnoxious parasite.

CANDIDA QUESTIONNAIRE*

If you suspect you might suffer from candidiasis, William Crook, MD, has developed a questionnaire that you can fill out to determine the likelihood. The score evaluation is at the end of the quiz.

SECTION ONE: History

There are different point scores for each question. Note the points and add them up.

QUESTIONS	POINTS
1. Have you taken tetracycline or other antibiotics for acne for one month or longer?	25
2. Have you at any time in your life taken other "broad-spectrum" antibiotics for respiratory, urinary, or other infections for two months or longer, or in short courses four or more times in a one-year period?	20
3. Have you ever taken a broad-spectrum antibiotic (even a single course)?	6
4. Have you at anytime in your	

*This questionnaire is adapted from William G. Crook, MD, *The Yeast Connection*. Although the Candida Questionnaire can help determine your condition, ultimately the best method for diagnosing candidiasis is clinical evaluation by a physician knowledgeable about yeast-related illness.

life been bothered by persistent
prostatitis, vaginitis, or other problems
affecting your reproductive organs? 25

5. Have you been pregnant one time? 3
Two or more times? 5

6. Have you taken birth control pills for
six months to two years? 8
For more than two years? 15

7. Have you taken prednisone or other
cortisone-type drugs for two weeks or less? 6
For more than two weeks? 15

8. Does exposure to perfumes,
insecticides, fabric shop odors, and
other chemicals provoke mild symptoms? 5
Moderate to severe symptoms? . 20

9. Are your symptoms worse on damp,
muggy days or in moldy places? 20

10. Have you had athlete's foot, ringworm,
jock itch, or other chronic infections
of the skin or nails?
Mild to moderate? 10
Severe or persistent? 20

11. Do you crave sugar? 10

12. Do you crave breads? 10

13. Do you crave alcoholic beverages? 10

14. Does tobacco smoke really bother you? 10

Total score for section one _____

SECTION TWO: **Major Symptoms**

For each of the symptoms below, enter the appropriate
score in the points column.

If a symptom is occasional or mild, score 3 points.

If a symptom is frequent and/or moderately severe, score
6 points.

If a symptom is severe and/or disabling, score 9 points.

SYMPTOMS	POINTS
1. Fatigue or lethargy	_____
2. Feeling of being drained	_____
3. Poor memory	_____
4. Feeling "spacey" or "unreal"	_____
5. Depression	_____
6. Numbness, burning, or tingling	_____
7. Muscle aches	_____
8. Muscle weakness or paralysis	_____
9. Pain and/or swelling in joints	_____
10. Abdominal pain	_____
11. Constipation	_____
12. Diarrhea	_____
13. Bloating	_____
14. Persistent vaginal itch	_____
15. Persistent vaginal burning	_____
16. Prostatitis	_____
17. Impotence	_____
18. Loss of sexual desire	_____

19. Endometriosis _____
20. Cramping and other menstrual irregularities_____
21. Premenstrual tension _____
22. Spots in front of eyes _____
23. Erratic vision _____

Total score for section two _____

SECTION THREE: Other Symptoms

For each of the symptoms below, enter the appropriate
score in the points column.

If a symptom is occasional or mild, score 1 point.

If a symptom is frequent and/or moderately severe, score
2 points.

If a symptom is severe and/or disabling, score 3 points.

SYMPTOMS	POINTS
1. Drowsiness	_____
2. Irritability	_____
3. Lack of coordination	_____
4. Inability to concentrate	_____
5. Frequent mood swings	_____
6. Headache	_____
7. Dizziness/loss of balance	_____
8. Pressure above ears, feeling of head swelling and tingling	_____
9. Itching	_____
10. Other rashes	_____

11. Heartburn   _____

12. Indigestion   _____

13. Belching and intestinal gas   _____

14. Mucus in stools   _____

15. Hemorrhoids   _____

16. Dry mouth   _____

17. Rash or blisters in mouth   _____

18. Bad breath   _____

19. Joint swelling or arthritis   _____

20. Nasal congestion or discharge   _____

21. Postnasal drip   _____

22. Nasal itching   _____

23. Sore or dry throat   _____

24. Cough   _____

25. Pain or tightness in chest   _____

26. Wheezing or shortness of breath   _____

27. Urinary urgency or frequency   _____

28. Burning on urination   _____

29. Failing vision   _____

30. Burning or tearing of eyes   _____

31. Recurrent infections or fluid in ears   _____

32. Ear pain or deafness   _____

Total score for section three   _____

Total score for section one   _____

Total score for section two   _____

Total score for section three   _____

Total score for all sections   _____

Results	Women	Men
Yeast-connected health problems are almost certainly present.	>180	>140
Yeast-connected health problems are probably present.	120–180	90–140
Yeast-connected health problems are possibly present.	60–119	40–89
Yeast-connected health problems are less likely to be present.	<60	<40

The Parasite Cleanse

Parasitic infestation is not limited to poor Third World countries, but is actually growing at an alarming rate right here in North America. A number of health care professionals believe parasites are the cause or a contributing factor to a number of disease conditions such as cancer and chronic fatigue.

A parasite is an organism that feeds off of another. In our bodies, parasites often feed on the undigested, putrefied food that collects in the gastrointestinal tract, the mucus of the lungs and lymphatic system, or any area of the body that is sick or weak, often because of toxic overload. These intruders are able to proliferate when the immune system is compromised. Although some parasites like worms are large enough to be visible in the stools, especially during a detoxification program when they are being expelled, most are microscopic pathogens that can be detected only by a specialized stool test.

Common sources of parasites include improperly washed vegetables and fruit, contaminated water, and undercooked meats. Parasites are often transmitted from pets and can be transferred from other infected persons. The overuse of antibiotics interferes with normal intestinal flora and contributes to parasites' proliferation.

Because parasites are difficult to detect and often hide in the lining of the intestinal tract or in other organs, their presence and the problems they cause may go undiagnosed or misdiagnosed. Parasites cause damage directly to the body, but also their acidic waste excretions contribute to additional body toxicity. Microscopic pathogens like yeasts, protozoa, fungi, and bacteria disrupt our digestive processes and contribute to compromised digestion, which negatively impacts the immune system and leads to compromised nutrition.

Parasites feed on the nutrients that are meant to nourish us. In other words, our cells may be starving because of the nutritional deficiencies that result from parasitic infestation. Often people with parasites will overeat, trying to make up for the nutritional deficit created by the parasites. If you suspect parasitic infestation, see your doctor or naturopath for a stool test (or you can order a test online; see the Resources Guide). However, if the parasites are localized in areas outside of the colon, such as the brain or lungs, these tests are often inconclusive.

Symptoms of Parasitic Infection

There's a huge variety of parasites and numerous diverse symptoms associated with them. Many of these symptoms are common for other conditions. See your doctor for a stool test to confirm the presence of parasites.

- Abdominal cramping and bloating
- Constipation
- Diarrhea
- Burning sensations when defecating
- Fluid loss
- Poor absorption of nutrients
- Irritable bowel syndrome
- Blood sugar fluctuations

- Food cravings
- Tiredness and weakness
- Allergies
- Anemia
- Fuzzy thinking
- Headaches
- Loose, foul-smelling stools
- Loss of appetite
- Coughing
- Fever
- Vomiting

The program that follows has been highly effective in helping many people rid themselves of these destructive pathogens.

EAT A WHOLE FOODS DIET

The standard American diet (SAD) of processed, high-carbohydrate foods, junk food, and nutrient-deficient fare contributes to parasitic infection by causing a buildup of wastes and toxins. Parasites love sugar and foods that quickly turn to sugar like pasta and bread, and the diet of most Americans is loaded with it. The detoxification programs in this book will help to cleanse and detoxify your colon, liver, gallbladder, kidneys, lymph, skin, and blood, which is an important step for parasite cleansing. You may need to continue with the Parasite Cleanse several weeks or months, as parasites can often be difficult to eliminate. Avoid the foods listed in the box below.

Foods to Avoid During a Parasite (or Candida) Cleanse

- All forms of sugars, even natural sugars like fruit—parasites feed on sugar
- Breads, pasta, flour products—these quickly turn to sugar and many contain yeast; avoid all products with yeast
- Milk and dairy products—these contain milk sugar
- Beer, wine, and all other alcoholic beverages—they turn to sugar and contain yeast
- Cheese—contains yeast and mold
- Dried fruit—contains sugar and mold
- Peanuts and peanut butter—these have a high mold content
- Mushrooms—a type of mold
- Coffee, tea, and tobacco—acquire molds or yeast in the drying process (exception: Pau D'Arco tea is helpful to kill off yeasts)

Your diet should include an abundance of beta-carotene-rich foods, which are converted to vitamin A as needed in the body. Vitamin A increases resistance to tissue penetration by parasitic larvae. Beta-carotene-rich foods include carrots, sweet potatoes, yams, squash, broccoli, parsley, kale, spinach, dandelion greens, and other dark leafy greens. These can be made into juices, or they can be eaten raw, slightly steamed, or baked.

Avoid foods that irritate the gastrointestinal tract or cause gas and bloating, which interferes with nutrient absorption. Diligently avoid overeating because it puts a strain on the entire digestive system, especially the colon and the liver. Many protein-rich foods like meat, fish, or even vegan foods such as beans, lentils, split peas, nuts, and seeds can cause irritation or flatulence. Limit gas-producing foods during the parasite cleanse. However, sprouted nuts, seeds, and beans are more easily digested and provide some protein. You may need to supplement your diet with natural free-form amino-acid protein powder during the cleanse. Gluten-containing grains such as wheat, rye, oats, and barley may cause irritation to the intestinal tract if you are gluten sensitive, and if that's true for you, should be avoided.

GARLIC

Garlic is a helpful treatment for the removal of parasites, especially common worms like roundworm, pinworm, and hookworm. Take two raw garlic cloves per day, finely minced. If you place it on a teaspoon and swallow with water without chewing, you won't taste it. Garlic is also available in capsules or tablets. The recommendation is 500 mg two to three times a day. Other helpful antiparasitic foods include onions, scallions, leeks, radish, kelp, raw cabbage, ground almonds, blackberries, pumpkin, sauerkraut, and fig extract.

HERBS

A variety of herbs are available to help kill and expel parasites and worms. Green/black walnut hull tincture is used for parasites in the blood as well as other parts of the body. For roundworms, the following combination of herbs is effective: green/black walnut hulls, wormwood, ground cloves, gentian root, ginger, and mandrake root. Pink root, also known as Indian Pink, was used by Native Americans to kill intestinal worms, especially roundworms. For removing flatworms such as tapes and flukes, the following combination of herbs is effective: male fern, pumpkin seeds, pink root, wood betony, chamomile, and senna. Other effective herbs include oil of oregano, artemisia, and cloves. Grapefruit-seed extract and enzymes such as bromelain, papain, and protease have been shown to also be helpful — the enzymes break through the mucus barrier that covers and protects the parasitic cysts. Grapefruit-seed extract has also been shown to eliminate protozoa and fungus on contact (found at health food stores).

AVOID ALL SUGARS

Sweets of all kinds, as well as sugar and sugar substitutes, should be avoided. As mentioned earlier, parasites love sugar and flourish on all forms of it. During your parasite detoxification it is imperative that you *do not eat any sweets.* Drinking a glass of water with lemon and a little stevia (herbal sweetener found at health food stores) can often satisfy the craving for sweets until you regain your will to resist.

CLEANSE THE INTESTINAL TRACT

Parasites cling to and feed off the mucus-encrusted layer in the intestinal tract. Therefore, your parasite detox will not be completely effective until the colon is thoroughly cleansed of this mucus layer. Otherwise, the parasites become embedded in this matter and hide out. Follow the Colon-Cleanse Program on pages 146–155 for at least two weeks before beginning the Parasite Cleanse. It's also helpful to complete the Liver/Gallbladder Detox before undertaking a parasite cleanse so all your principal organs of elimination are functioning optimally.

DIGESTIVE AND SYSTEMIC ENZYMES

Digestive enzymes are necessary for the proper digestion of food. Unless your diet is primarily raw food, your natural enzyme levels may be insufficient for optimum digestion, so a good enzyme supplement will aid digestion and relieve the body of some of its burden of enzyme production.

Digestive enzymes are taken with meals to help digest protein, carbs, and fat. Protease, lipase, amylase, bromelain, and papain are examples of supplemental digestive enzymes. Systemic enzymes are different from digestive enzymes in that they are taken between meals, usually about two hours after eating, to clean up undigested proteins and help maintain healthy blood and tissue functions. (See the Resources Guide for systemic enzymes.)

The Thirty-Day Heavy-Metal Detoxification Program

Living in the twenty-first century exposes every one of us to contamination from heavy metals. These intoxicants pour into our environment from hundreds of sources that contaminate our air, water, food, buildings, and gardens. Lead is a common heavy metal that has been in our environment for decades. It's found in the solder that seals food cans, in crops grown in lead-contaminated soil, in atmospheric lead from glass manufacturers, from printers, smelters, and various other sources of industrial lead, as well as from leaded dust that is used in ceramic glazes. Although gas and paint no longer contain lead, many of us who grew up in that era still have lead in our tissues from exposure during the 1950s, '60s, and '70s.

Mercury levels have become so high in many of our oceans and lakes that it has contaminated much of the world's fish and shellfish. The mercury becomes more concentrated as you move up the food chain, so larger fish like albacore tuna, swordfish, and shark are often highly contaminated. Fish meal is frequently fed to chickens (unless they're fed a vegan diet), so poultry is an additional source of mercury. Another common source is dental fillings, which are an amalgam of mercury and silver, as well as from vaccinations that can contain the compound thimerosal (mercury is used as a preservative). We are exposed to cadmium from phosphate fertilizers, the burning of fossil fuels, and the gases that are released from zinc, lead, and copper smelters. Tobacco smoke is also a source of cadmium. Other types of heavy metals that may accumulate in our bodies from environmental pollution include arsenic, tin, copper, and aluminum. Heavy metals tend to accumulate in the tissues of the brain, kidneys, liver, fat cells, and immune system. They are not easily eliminated by the normal channels of elimination, but tend to stay in our bodies for decades, often severely disrupting normal metabolic function and sometimes causing irreversible damage. Their effects can range from subtle symptoms to serious diseases, and because metals build up in the body over long periods of time, the associated symptoms are often misdiagnosed.

Removal of heavy metals can be a slow, difficult process, and during a detoxification program there is usually a redistribution of heavy metals within the body. To rid yourself of them, carefully follow the guidelines in this section during your detoxification program.

Symptoms of Heavy Metal Toxicity

- Chronic pain in muscles and tendons or any soft tissues of the body
- Chronic fatigue
- Malaise—a general feeling of discontent, fatigue, illness, and lethargy
- Brain fog—state of forgetfulness and confusion
- Chronic infections such as *Candida albicans*
- Gastrointestinal disturbance such as diarrhea, constipation, bloating, gas, heartburn, and indigestion
- Food allergies and intolerances
- Dizziness
- Migraines or headaches
- Visual problems
- Mood swings, depression, and anxiety
- Nervous system malfunctions—burning extremities, numbness, tingling, paralysis, or an electrifying feeling throughout the body

Because heavy metal toxicity can produce symptoms that sometimes are mistaken for other chronic conditions such as chronic fatigue syndrome, depression, or multiple sclerosis, it's wise to discuss heavy metal toxicity with a qualified health-care professional.

EAT AN ALKALINE DIET

Step 1 of our cleansing program outlines the principles of an alkaline diet. It's extremely important during a heavy-metal detox that you eat a diet that is 70 to 85 percent alkaline (see box "Acid Versus Alkaline Foods" on page 23). Include a variety of the cruciferous vegetables such as broccoli, kale, cabbage, cauliflower, Brussels sprouts, as well as plenty of dark, leafy green vegetables to provide extra minerals and calcium. Heavy metals can displace vitamins and minerals, so continue with your daily juicing.

Unlike most of the other detoxification programs, you'll want to consume adequate amounts of protein. Consume two to three grams of meat or fish once or twice a day. Choose grass-fed beef, organic free-range poultry and eggs, or wild-caught fish. Alternatively, you can use vegan protein such as beans, lentils, split peas, whole grains (exclude wheat), nuts, and seeds, either raw or sprouted. A heavy-metal detox is not the time for a fast. You need plenty of amino acids during this time. One reason is for the production of the antioxidant glutathione, a tripeptide (three amino acids linked together) that is important in liver detoxification and greatly facilitates the removal of heavy metals. The other important reason for adequate protein consumption is that amino acids bind to heavy metals, and fasting can break down protective protein layers, exposing metals, causing damage in the absence of adequate protein. A protein powder supplement may be beneficial.

DRINK PLENTY OF CARROT JUICE

Carrot juice contains vitamins, minerals, and phytochemicals that are especially needed as antioxidants during heavy-metal detoxification. Drink two glasses of carrot juice each day; you may add celery, cucumber, parsley, sprouts, jicama, any greens such as kale, spinach, beet leaves, and flavor with ginger, or herbs such as cilantro.

CILANTRO, GARLIC, CHLORELLA, AND CHLOROPHYLL

Cilantro has been demonstrated to aid in the removal of heavy metals from the body. Add it to salads, soups, juices, and salsas. Sulfur-containing foods such as garlic and onions also help to combat heavy-metal toxicity. Chlorophyll and chlorella are also known to aid in heavy-metal detoxification. Use concentrated greens products, liquid chlorophyll, or chlorella.

WATER

Drink eight to ten 8-ounce glasses (2 to 2 1/2 quarts) of purified water each day; alkalinizing water is quite beneficial.

SUPPLEMENT WITH FIBER SHAKES

Drink one to two fiber shakes each day. You can make your own (see page 151 in chapter five on colon cleansing) or purchase a commercial blend. It's also advisable to take an herbal formula once or twice daily. (These must be purchased. See Resources Guide for recommendations.) The fiber will help to absorb the metals, preventing them from being reabsorbed back into the system.

DO NOT TAKE ENZYMES DURING THIS CLEANSE

Enzymes can remove the protein that carries heavy metals out of the body, exposing the metals and causing damage.

SUPPLEMENTS AFTER MEALS

Probiotic formula: two after each meal (a friendly-bacteria formula).

REMOVE MERCURY AMALGAM FILLINGS

Silver dental fillings are made from an amalgam of mercury and silver. The mercury can be released as a vapor during chewing or cleaning your teeth. The resultant release of mercury causes it to be deposited in tissues throughout the body. Mercury from dental fillings is one of the principal contributors to human exposure to inorganic mercury. Studies have shown that people with mercury-containing dental fillings show an association between the number and size of the fillings and the amount of mercury found in their urine.

IMMUNIZATIONS AND MERCURY

Thimerosal is a preservative that is still used in a number of vaccines. It contains 49 percent ethyl mercury by weight and generally contributes to as much as 25 mcg of ethyl mercury per dose. For decades mercury-containing vaccinations were given to infants on a regular basis. However, because of the danger to health, the Food and Drug Administration has recently recommended that thimerosal be removed from all pediatric vaccines. (It may still be in some; check with your physician.) Nevertheless, it is still routinely used in influenza vaccines. Some scientists believe that past indiscriminate use of thimerosal-containing vaccinations is related to the growing U.S. epidemic of autism. Before you get a vaccine or allow your children to be vaccinated, make sure the vaccine contains no thimerosal or any other mercury-containing compound.

DETOX REACTIONS IN THE HEAVY-METAL CLEANSE

The Thirty-Day Heavy-Metal Detoxification Program can initiate cold or flu symptoms or other distressing reactions like headaches. Cleansing reactions usually last only a few days. The presence of detox symptoms simply means the process is working, so don't be alarmed or deterred. Soon the symptoms will pass as the toxins are eliminated and health is restored.

CHAPTER EIGHT

Mental and Emotional Cleansing

The last phase of your program is mental and emotional cleansing. A juice fast or colon cleanse will certainly detox and renew your body, but any physical cleanse will be greatly enhanced by also detoxing your mind and emotions. How many people do you know who are worried, fearful, anxious, pessimistic, irritated, or critical? Maybe some of these responses apply to you. It's a stressful world that we live in and it's difficult to avoid negative thinking. But there's a price to pay for these thoughts and emotions that don't serve us. We can learn how to replace them with positive, health-enhancing thoughts and emotions that contribute to our well-being.

Mental and emotional toxicity leads to chemical toxicity in the body and can have devastating physical effects. For example, unresolved issues, defeating toxic thoughts, and emotional baggage are often contributing factors to a variety of physical symptoms such as migraine headaches, fatigue, fibromyalgia, insomnia, multiple chemical sensitivities, poor immune response, and intestinal problems. Research also links toxic thoughts and emotions to serious illnesses such as cancer and heart disease, as well as to anxiety, panic attacks, and depression.

Cleansing these thoughts and emotions from our body and soul is as important to our health as detoxing pesticides and industrial chemicals from our tissues. "If we don't root them out, they can become imbedded in the soul," says best-selling author Dr. Christiane Northrup. "A thought held long enough and repeated often enough becomes a belief." And that belief causes a biological change in the body. For example, stress causes the adrenal glands to produce corticosteroids — hormones that weaken the immune system, glandular function, and other systems. Suppressed anger is one of the most toxic emotional responses of all and leads to chronic ill health and poor behavioral choices.

When we can rid our lives of negativity, we can begin to create the health and life we want. To cleanse toxic thoughts and emotions we need both mental and physical action that can transform the effects of unhealthy neurochemicals that have built up in our body.

The Hard Facts on Toxic Thinking and Its Effects on the Body

What we focus on mentally and emotionally becomes our experience. We may have entertained negative thoughts such as irritation, resentment, criticism, and judgment of others and ourselves for years and, consequently, they have become so habitual that we are unaware of them. They may even seem "normal," but negative thinking is not normal; it's physically destructive. Negative emotions like anger, hate, worry, fear, jealousy, irritation, and bitterness can make us sick and pave the way to life-threatening diseases. These emotions are transmitted to the entire body through neurons and neuropeptides that send messages for good or for ill.

Candace Pert, PhD, one of the foremost neurobiologists of our time and former chief of brain chemistry at the National Institute of Mental Health, has written extensively about the connection between emotions and neuropeptides. She and her husband discovered that neuropeptides, which are chemicals that affect mood and behavior, join the brain, glands, and immune system in a network of communication that can affect us on a cellular level.

Here's how it works: White blood cells have receptor sites for neuropeptides, and when our thoughts are negative, the messengers' (neuropeptides) communication can disrupt the health of our immune cells. Negative thoughts and emotions have been found to decrease T cell production and activity and to release stress hormones. Some neuropeptides can even trigger cancer cells to metastasize. Conversely, others help keep our body healthy.

Chemicals produced by toxic emotions lodge in our muscles and we can experience neck and back pain or pain in other parts of our body. We can experience weakness, intestinal disturbances such as constipation, headaches, and depression. The effects of negative emotions are also stored in the liver and kidneys and can disrupt their function and block proper pancreatic function. Unhealthy emotions can also cause cognitive inhibition, affecting our ability to comprehend, think, and make rational decisions. And traumatic memories may trigger allergic reactions. The list could go on and on, but the point to remember is that negative emotions are disruptive to the body, produce toxicity, and can be devastating to our health.

The Mind-Body Connection

The mind-body connection, meaning the connection between thinking, emotions, and the health of the body, is not new. But we forget how powerful this connection is. There are distinct emotional and mental patterns associated with illness. The way you choose to use your mind, will, and emotions and the way you respond to your outer world has as much, if not more, to do with disease as your diet, lifestyle, and environment.

The body is a mirror of your inner thoughts, emotions, and beliefs. Every cell in your body has its own intelligence and is able to listen to what you are thinking and feel what you are expressing. Your cells respond to each thought, every emotion, and every word you say. Repetitive methods of negative thinking and suppressing negative emotions such as anger, resentment, and hatred, and even those that seem milder such as irritation, annoyance, or frustration, can eventually manifest as illness. Negative thinking is like a ticking bomb waiting for the perfect conditions to explode.

Science has shown that when you are in a state of distress, your cells come into disharmony. When you operate in stress and negative thinking, toxic chemicals are created, which promotes sick cells. Once you are in this state, you are prone to attracting viruses, harmful bacteria, parasites, and *Candida albicans* (yeast).

More than any other factor, emotional stress weakens the immune system, and you are less able to control everything from parasites to cancer cells. Also, when you are stressed or harboring unhealthy emotions, you tense up. This tension causes biological processes to be impaired. Nutrient transport, cell respiration, detoxification, elimination, digestion, assimilation, hormone production, and brain function become disrupted leading to a gradual degeneration in the body. But when you are in a state of balance — mentally, emotionally, spiritually, and physically — illness simply can't settle in your body.

Most people have not been taught how to deal with stress or negative thinking, and don't know how to live a balanced life. Our society promotes drama, tension, stress, negativity, and struggle, which makes natural, relaxed behavior nearly impossible. The secret to being free of the effects of all these unhealthy responses is to stop thinking, suppressing, and storing negative thoughts and emotions, find your divine purpose, learn to love all creatures, and live your life in a positive, joy-filled expression of who you really are.

Transforming Toxic Thoughts

By detoxifying your physical body, you begin a process that will help you cleanse and transform your thoughts and emotions. As you pour fresh live juices and veggie smoothies into your body, they will push out toxic substances that have been stored in tissues, fluids, and cells. Emotions attached to toxic substances often surface when you cleanse. You can assist this process by allowing old thought patterns and emotions to come into full consciousness during detoxification and then release them and let them go. You may need to "dig up" others and release them so you can be free.

The first step in the process of letting go is to identify unhealthy thoughts. You may not be aware that some of your thinking, which may seem quite routine and normal, is actually toxic. You may have grown up in a negative family, and such thinking seems routine. Or maybe you've just thought critically or pessimistically for years because of circumstances in your life. This is not normal. Loving and positive thoughts are normal. Daily examination of your thinking is a process that can help you root out these thoughts and replace them with positive life-giving words.

Examples of negative thinking follow. Place a check by those that apply to you and add to the list as similar unproductive thoughts come to mind.

_____ I hate my body.
_____ I'm too short, too fat, too skinny.
_____ I hate my nose.
_____ My hair is too curly, too straight, too fine.
_____ I'm ugly.
_____ I hate my thighs.
_____ I can't stand my life.
_____ My children don't love me.
_____ Nobody loves me.
_____ I'm never going to find a job I enjoy.

_____ I don't know if I'll ever find the right person to spend my life with.

_____ I'm never going to get well.

_____ I have an incurable disease.

_____ Nobody cares about me.

_____ I had a terrible childhood.

_____ I have a rotten marriage.

_____ I can't stand my job.

_____ There's never enough money to pay my bills.

_____ My life has no meaning or purpose.

_____ I'm lonely.

_____ I don't like where I live.

_____ I've never done anything exciting in my life.

_____ My mother/father treated me terribly.

_____ Nothing ever works out for me.

_____ I've always had a poor immune system.

_____ My life will never change.

This list could go on and on. The important thing is to do some self-assessment and recognize when your thoughts are either life enhancing or self-defeating. Your inner dialogue promotes health or dis-ease. That's why it's so important to root out destructive thinking. For each negative thought you checked off on this list, you can practice letting it go. (See pages 248–254 for the letting go exercises.)

Become aware of when you think negative thoughts. Here are some examples of how you can transform destructive, self-defeating thinking into positive thoughts. The next time a negative thought comes to mind such as "I hate my life," you can choose to think, "I'm working on finding my purpose, which is life-giving." If you think, "I'm never going to find a job I enjoy," you can say, "The right job awaits me; someone needs my skills and talents." If you think about your poor health and are tempted to think you'll never be healthy and full of life again, you can choose to think, "The juicing and cleansing I'm doing and all the good choices I'm making will produce better health. I'm getting better and healthier every day." Intercept all negativity as soon as it pops into your mind. You can say something like, "I cancel that thought" or whatever you choose to keep your mind from dwelling on this kind of thinking. As you practice this daily, you'll build a new habit of positive thinking.

Transforming Toxic Emotions

The word "emotion" literally means "energy in motion." It's derived from a Latin verb meaning "to move." An emotion is a strong feeling such as love, fear, sorrow, or anger. Emotions move us; they generate complex mental and physiological reactions that produce change and affect our health on a cellular level. Emotional experiences get imprinted in brain cells, as well as cells throughout the body, where they form patterns that influence our behavior and the chemistry of our bodies.

Emotional energy functions at a higher speed than thought. Scientists have confirmed that emotional reactions are recorded in brain activity before we even have time to think about them. We evaluate everything on an emotional level, and afterward, we think about it.

Being in touch with our emotions and learning to channel them in healthy ways, rather than stuff them or express them inappropriately, will lead to greater cellular and system health in our bodies.

Pure emotions such as anger or fear are not good or bad in themselves. We all need to feel fear so that we won't walk out in front of an oncoming car or wait too long to light a gas stove or fireplace. Sometimes we need to feel anger so that we can rise to the defense of someone or something in need, such as a child being abused, an animal being mistreated, or a country being torn apart. But we also need to let emotions go that don't serve us, such as bitterness, resentment, blame, or irritation; they are never pure and always toxic.

Repressed traumas, which cause overwhelming

emotions, can get stored for years in cells, tissues, and organs, thereby affecting their function. Trauma produces intense emotions that can become stuck in cells and cause breaks in being. Much has been written about sexual abuse and the traumatizing effects it continues to have on people who were molested as children. The same goes for physical abuse, verbal abuse, neglect, abandonment, isolation, rape, and many other traumas. What we know is that any form of trauma, whether emotional or physical, is stored in the body. When these traumas happen to children, they are stored in the child's body and can cause the child to grow up with unhealed memories, pent-up emotions, and imbalanced neurotransmitters. And whether the trauma happened in childhood or as an adult, unless dealt with, cleansed, and let go of, the traumas can be like ticking time bombs, just waiting for the right moment to explode. Holding on to events and unhealthy emotions creates problems because they are stored on the cellular level. They need to be released for our well-being.

Releasing unhealthy emotional energy is essential for our cleansing process. Love, forgiveness, and letting go of demands that things in our life be different are keys to neutralizing the effects of toxic emotions in our bodies. This can facilitate the cleansing process, promote physical health, and lead to joy and wholeness.

Toxic Emotions: Contributors to Disease

Anguish	Grief	Sorrow
Anxiety	Guilt	Strife
Bitterness	Hate	Unforgiveness
Blame	Humiliation	Unhealthy or
Confusion	Insecurity	suppressed
Defilement	Irritation	anger
Despair	Rage	Worry
Discouragement	Rejection of self	Worthlessness
Envy	Resentment	Wrath
Fear (unhealthy)	Shame	

Cleansing Negative Emotions: The Letting Go Method

The "Sedona Method," also called the "Release Technique," is a simple, yet powerful process that helps us release unwanted emotions that may be poisoning our body and soul.

The creator of this method, Lester Levenson, nearly died of a massive heart attack and was given just weeks to live by his physicians. During an intense period of self-examination, he came to believe that it was not the world or the people in it that were the cause of his problems. He acknowledged that his own emotional responses to events in his life had caused his health issues. Levenson discovered that he was capable of completely discharging all his negative emotions. As a result his health and life flourished, and the Sedona Method was born.

This technique has undergone numerous scientific studies. Dr. Richard Davidson of the Laboratory of Cognitive Psychobiology at the State University of New York, and Dr. David McClelland of the Department of Psychology and Social Relations at Harvard University conducted one such study. They concluded that the Sedona Method was highly effective in stress reduction. In a three-and-a-half-month follow-up study, dramatic reductions in stress were still present for participants.

Levenson found that people have three ways in which they deal with a feeling — they *suppress* it, they *express* it, or they *escape.*

When feelings are *suppressed*, we create an environment in which tension, anxiety, and depression can fester. This is very toxic to the body, and the most harmful way to deal with the emotions. Suppressed emotions create physical problems and behavior that is very unhealthy and sometimes uncontrollable.

Some people deal with emotions by expressing or venting them often. But even when an emotion is vented, it doesn't go away; it still needs to be dealt with. And after a blowup, there's often an accompanying emotion of guilt. We are usually remorseful for our lack of control, and, often, for the unkind words we spoke. All in all, expressing negative emotions is not a healthy way to deal with them either.

The third way people deal with their emotions is to escape, which may be watching television, reading a book, surfing the Internet, eating, calling a friend, shopping, drinking alcohol, gambling, using recreational or prescription drugs, having sex, or smoking. But the emotions that are causing stress in the body are still there. Like the other two ways of dealing with emotions, escape does not work.

There is a healthy way to deal with our emotions. Many great teachers have taught this way throughout time. *Release* the feeling — simply *let it go.* (The technique follows.) Discharging the feeling is the healthiest way to deal with emotions. Laughter is one form of release. Most of us have had arguments in which, all of a sudden, we realize how silly the whole thing is and burst into laughter. At that point our bodies feel light and free. The emotion released was no longer in the body's tissues or contaminating our dialogue.

When we put the release technique into practice it has a cumulative effect. We become more clearheaded, more productive, and calm. Over time we can reach a state of imperturbability in which nothing can throw us off center. We can maintain our "cool" whatever the situation. We become more productive on the job, happier in our relationships, and at peace with our life.

Here's how the technique is completed:

STEP 1: FOCUS

Select a problem area in your life. Choose something with a lot of "emotional charge." Now, allow yourself to become relaxed and calm.

STEP 2: FEEL THE EMOTION

Ask yourself, "What am I feeling right now?" It really is important to tell the truth about your feelings. Listed below are six primary toxic emotions with many other emotions that are associated in those six categories. Identify the ones that apply to you.

Anger: Associated emotions that fall under anger are rage, aggression, annoyance, argumentative, defiant, demanding, disgusted, irritated, frustrated, furious, hateful, impatient, jealous, mad, mean, outraged, resentful, spiteful, stubborn, sullen, vengeful, vicious, and violent.

Apathy: Associated emotions that fall under the category of apathy are bored, careless, defeated, depressed, discouraged, disillusioned, drained, futile, hopeless, overwhelmed, powerless, resigned, and worthless.

Fear: Feelings subtyped under fear include anxious, apprehensive, cautious, cowardly, doubtful, dreadful, foreboding, inhibited, insecure, nervous, panicky, scared, shaky, trapped, and worried.

Grief: Some subtypes of grief are feelings of abandonment, abuse, accused, anguish, ashamed, betrayed, cheated, embarrassed, helpless, hurt, ignored, left out, misunderstood, neglected, rejected, and sad.

Lust: This emotion of lust yells "I want" and subtypes include anticipation, craving, demanding, desiring, devious, driven, envious, frustrated, greedy, manipulative, obsessed, ruthless, selfish, and wicked.

Pride: Some associated feelings under pride are aloof, arrogant, boastful, clever, contemptuous, cool, critical, judgmental, self-righteous, rigid, self-satisfied, snobbish, spoiled, superior, selfish, unforgiving, and vain.

STEP 3: IDENTIFY YOUR FEELING

Focus on what you are feeling at this time as you think about what has caused you hurt, fear, loss, rejection, or any other harmful response to an offense. Watch your body and identify what it's doing. Is your heart beating quickly? Are your eyes tearing? Do you feel nauseous? Is there tension in your muscles? Whatever is happening in your body is a clue to the emotions that need to be released.

Now select a word that best describes your feeling. When you have selected the word, find it in one of the six root-word categories. The process of release is most effective when the root emotion is released in its purest form along with all associated emotions. For example, it's more effective to release anger than it is to release the emotion of being annoyed. It's like pulling a weed out by its roots, rather than just cutting back the plant. When the root has been removed, the weed is gone for good.

STEP 4: FEEL YOUR FEELING

Allow yourself to experience your emotions. Perhaps you feel angry. Allow yourself to be angry. Or perhaps you feel grief or sorrow. Allow yourself to be sad or to grieve. You may find yourself crying or sobbing. That is exactly what needs to happen at this time. It's okay to allow your feelings to permeate your body. This is not the time to stuff emotions or shut them down.

STEP 5: COULD YOU LET GO?

While you are feeling the feeling, ask yourself the simple question "Could I let this feeling go?" One of the most freeing aspects of being an adult is being able to differentiate between our emotions and our true self. That means that our emotions aren't us. They are simply energy moving through our bodies. Each of us has a "watcher or true self" that can observe the emotions as they flow through the body. It's this watcher that is asking the question, "Could I let go of this feeling?" We can view the emotion as a shadow image that has superimposed itself over who we really are. The feeling is not who we are, even though it may seem overwhelming.

Once we realize that we can feel the feeling and our true self can ask a question at the very same time, we are able to see the possibility of letting the feeling go.

STEP 6: WOULD YOU LET IT GO?

Once we realize that we can let the feeling go, it's possible for us to release it. We can ask ourselves, "Would I let it go?" This is where we need to be very honest. Sometimes we are simply too angry, hurt, or afraid to let it go at the present time. In that case we need to allow ourselves to continue feeling our feelings and not intellectualize or escape from them. There will come a time when we're ready to let the emotions go. We'll eventually get fed up with the effect they are having on our bodies, of the mind chatter, and of the disharmony they cause in our lives. When this happens we can truly say from the heart, "Yes, I can let this feeling go."

We may also answer no. Whatever you answer is okay; just repeat the process every so often until the answer is yes.

STEP 7: WHEN WILL YOU LET IT GO?

Once we have acknowledged the possibility of letting this feeling go, the next question is, "When?" Am I ready to let it go now, in ten minutes, tomorrow, next week? When will I let this feeling go? There will come a point when the answer is, "Now! I'm willing to let this feeling go now. Right now! I don't want it anymore. I've processed this enough. I don't want to feel like this anymore. I want to be free."

STEP 8: RELEASE

Once the decision has been made to let it go, the next step is simply to release it — let it go. You could picture it flying away like a dove or drifting off like balloons. Releasing your emotions will bring a wave of relief to your body. You may find yourself laughing, crying, or perceiving a sensation of chills going up and down your spine. Whatever the sensation, you'll feel lighter, as if a heavy burden has just been lifted from your body.

STEP 9: REPEAT

Once you have released the feeling, it's time to observe your body. You may find that there are other emotions that need to be released. Simply go through the process as many times as needed. It's like peeling an onion. When one layer is gone, you may find that there's more to peel. Be patient with yourself and continue. It may take a period of time to completely cleanse your body and soul of all destructive emotions. Don't give up. This process works and creates a clean slate for you to begin the next phase in your cleansing and healing process.

Most people who use this technique find that their energy skyrockets, their bodies are less tense, and they are more at peace with themselves and the world. The more the technique is used, the easier it becomes. People who practice this technique find that they are able to release emotions as they arise, making their family life or work environment much more congenial and peaceful.

THE FINAL STEP

The more you practice the release technique, the more aware you may become of an underlying discontent and that you *want* more and more. There are two basic layers of want — wanting *approval* or wanting *control.* Until these underlying wants are released, there is always going to be an inner state of discontentment. The want to control or the want for approval will continue to underlie our emotions until they are released. When we release them, we'll have a wonderful sense of freedom!

The Highest State of Being

The state of imperturbability is one of the highest states we can attain. This is a state where toxic emotions like irritation, resentment, bitterness, and worry are not allowed to remain in our consciousness. We can be in a place of serenity and peace all the time, a place where nothing can throw us off our course or hinder our journey toward wholeness. This is the state where our bodies can mend and heal from illness or disease, where we can conquer addictions and make life-giving choices consistently.

Forgiveness

Forgiveness is healing for body and soul, whereas, unforgiveness and an unforgiving spirit are detrimental to our health. Unforgiveness can lead to immune suppression and a host of diseases and it can block the flow of energy in our bodies. Blocked or stagnant energy drains the body and taxes the immune system. When we hang on to unforgiveness, we hold ourselves in bondage. Though we may hold out on forgiving someone because we believe the wrongdoer must pay, and we'll not let him or her go in our minds and hearts until there is justice, it's our own bodies that pay the price and we are wounded all over again.

At times we may feel as if we're in control when we hold a grudge and unforgiveness in our heart. We may be tempted to think that this can defend against the hurt, disappointment, or anger we feel about what was done to us, but the truth is that unforgiveness and attempting to control another person or situation actually makes us powerless and we are hurt in the end. A rattlesnake, if cornered, will sometimes become so angry it will bite itself. That is exactly what harboring unforgiveness and corresponding toxic emotions such as hate, resentment, or bitterness is like — a biting and poisoning of oneself. We may think that we're giving the person what they deserve by holding spite, but the deeper harm is to ourselves. Just how often should we forgive? As often as we experience unforgiveness. The "seventy times seven" admonition concerning forgiveness is an Eastern idiom for infinite forgiveness.

Forgiveness and healing are linked. Forgiveness is the antidote to the emotional poison of the soul. Just as fiber carries waste out of the colon, forgiveness carries emotional toxicity out of our soul. Where hatred is a roadblock to health, forgiveness is the bridge to life and healing. For forgiveness to be complete and unconditional, we must be willing to let go of all stored emotions such as bitterness, blame, grief, animosity, resentment, anger, irritation, or any other toxic emotion and forgive from the heart.

Forgiveness: A Key to Releasing Harmful Emotions

When we forgive others from our heart, not just our head, we free ourselves. In forgiveness, we're less driven to get even or to harm the one who hurt us. Forgiveness is positively linked to mental health and well-being. People who regularly forgive others report less depression, hostility, and anger. They are more hopeful and show higher self-esteem. Studies have shown that forgiving an offender leads to more positive emotions and a greater sense of control in one's life. In 2001, Charlotte van Oyen Witvliet and colleagues tested the physiological responses of undergraduates as they imagined real-life offenders in both forgiving and unforgiving ways. During forgiveness sessions, they empathized with the humanity of their offender and forgave the person. After the sessions, they reported less physiological stress, fewer negative emotions, more positive emotions, and a greater sense of control. The study found that empathy for the transgressor was a prevailing route to forgiveness.

To transform the emotions that have resulted from hurtful situations, and thus the memory of the hurt we've experienced, it can be helpful to go through some steps of forgiveness. You could address the following questions:

1. What do you know about the past of the person who hurt you? What was childhood like for the offender? Can you name a few things that could have contributed to this person's vulnerability? Remember that forgiving does not mean excusing someone's behavior. Also, make sure this person's hardships don't become your own.

2. At the time of the hurtful offense, what was life like for this person? Think about what he or she might have been thinking or feeling at this time. Was there a lot of pressure in this person's life? Was he or she feeling vulnerable?

3. What was your relationship with this person before the offense? How long had you known the person? Did you share any good times together? Name three positive things about this person.

4. As a result of the hurtful event, how might the offender be worse off now than before? What do you think life is like for him or her since the offense?

5. This person is a member of the human community. Though you do not need to welcome this person back into your life, can you see this person as part of the human family?

6. Has your view of this person changed in any way since answering these questions? Is there anything you can do to broaden your view of this person?

7. Can you let go of the offense and forgive this person?

CHAPTER NINE

The A to Z Guide to the Nutrient Content of Foods

The following lists show the nutrient content of various foods. These lists can be used as a guide in planning your menu choices so you can meet your nutritional needs with food. As you read through the lists, note the various foods that you may not eat on a regular basis, but that are high in certain nutrients. One of the best ways to ensure that you are getting your daily requirements of vitamins and minerals is to eat a variety of different foods. Try to add something new to your menu every day. Most of the vegetables can be juiced (unless they are dense like avocados). Juicing further concentrates the nutrients and is a great way to obtain value from vegetables you might not normally consume, such as kale, Swiss chard, beet greens, or turnip greens. Combine these green leafy vegetables with carrots, beets, cucumber, or celery and add some lemon, lime, green apple, or ginger for better-tasting juice.

While the values given in these lists can be useful in comparing the nutrient content of foods, absolute values for food nutrients will vary depending on such factors as the condition of the soil, type of fertilization, where the food was grown, how it was grown, the amount of processing or refining, and the method of preparation (cooked versus raw).

Keep in mind that studies show organic foods have a higher nutrient content and much less toxic contamination (especially from pesticides) than conventionally grown foods. Avoid genetically modified (GM or GMO) foods. Be especially mindful of soybeans and corn, and products made from them, as the majority of these crops are now GMO. Choose organically grown, as they are by definition non-GMO.

If you have questions about how to increase certain nutrients like vitamin C, potassium, calcium, or zinc, this guide provides valuable information to help you make wise choices. Some of the highest sources of these important nutrients are not widely known. For instance, almost everyone thinks that oranges and orange juice are among the best sources of vitamin C, yet vegetable sources like red peppers contain five times more vitamin C than oranges, and without the high fruit sugar. Another common example is the potassium content of bananas. For decades bananas have been advertised as one of the best sources of potassium, whereas vegetable sources like avocados, parsley, spinach, and Swiss chard are much richer in this mineral; and sunflower seeds and almonds contain almost twice the potassium as bananas. Instead of using whole milk for calcium, try some of the vegetable sources like kale, parsley, collard greens, and turnip greens — gram for gram these contain about twice the calcium as milk.

When choosing seafood, keep in mind that many of our oceans are contaminated with various toxins, notably heavy metals like mercury. Shellfish such as shrimp, crab, oysters, lobster, muscles, clams, and scallops are high in various nutrients, especially many of the minerals; however, these shellfish are also frequently contaminated with toxins, particularly because they are bottom feeders that clean up garbage in the ocean. So be mindful of overconsumption of seafood. Additionally, be aware that mercury and other heavy metals tend to accumulate in larger fish because they are higher up on the food chain and heavy metals stay in their tissues. Eat sparingly of swordfish, albacore tuna, and shark. A safer alternative is to substitute smaller fish like trout, sardines, or salmon (wild-caught only). Use wisdom in all your food choices, balancing the nutrient values with awareness of the possible contamination from the many sources of toxicity in our environment.

How to Use This Guide*

The quantity of each food on the lists, which have been developed by the U.S. Department of Agriculture, has been standardized to 100 grams instead of reporting them in common measurements. This provides a more appropriate comparison between relative amounts of nutrients in foods and allows them to be ranked from highest to lowest. Remember that not all foods are consumed in 100-gram quantities as they may be very concentrated, such as kelp, dulse, wheat germ, and brewer's yeast. These foods often appear at the top of the list indicating them as concentrated nutrient sources. The following conversions may be useful to give you a better idea of what 100 grams of a food represents in common measurements.

APPROXIMATE EQUIVALENTS

I teaspoon fluid	= about 5 grams
I teaspoon dry	= about 4 grams
I cup milk, yogurt	= 245 grams
I cup leafy vegetable	= 90 grams
I cup root vegetable	= 135 grams
I cup nuts, seeds	= 140 grams
I cup sliced fruit	= 150 grams
I cup cereal grain, uncooked	= 200 grams
I tablespoon cooking oil	= 14 grams
I tablespoon honey, molasses	= 20 grams

*This list was developed by the U.S. Department of Agriculture.

The Order of This Guide

VITAMINS

- Vitamin A
- Vitamin B complex
  - B1 thiamin
  - B2 riboflavin
  - B3 niacin
  - B5 pantothenic acid
  - B6 pyridoxine
  - B7 biotin
  - B9 folic acid
  - B10 PABA
  - B12 cyanocobalamin
  - B15 pangamic acid
  - B17 amygdalin (sometimes called laetrile)
  - choline
  - inositol
- Vitamin C ascorbic acid
  - Bioflavonoids
- Vitamin D
- Vitamin E
- Vitamin K

MINERALS

- Calcium
- Chromium
- Copper
- Iodine
- Iron
- Magnesium
- Manganese
- Molybdenum
- Nickel
- Phosphorus
- Potassium
- Selenium
- Sodium
- Vanadium
- Zinc

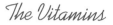

The Vitamins

Vitamin A

IU per 100 grams edible portion (100 grams = 3 1/2 ounces)

21,600 Peppers, red chili	2,000 Green onions
14,000 Dandelion greens	1,900 Romaine lettuce
11,000 Carrots	1,750 Papayas
10,900 Apricots, dried	1,650 Nectarines, prunes
9,300 Collard greens	1,600 Pumpkin
8,900 Kale	1,330 Peaches
8,800 Sweet potatoes	1,200 Acorn squash
8,500 Parsley	1,180 Eggs
8,100 Spinach	1,080 Chicken
7,600 Turnip greens	1,000 Cherries, sour red
7,000 Mustard greens	970 Butterhead lettuce
6,500 Swiss chard	900 Asparagus
6,100 Beet greens	900 Peppers, green chili
5,800 Chives	900 Tomatoes, ripe
5,700 Butternut squash	690 Kidneys
4,900 Watercress	640 Green peas
4,800 Mangos	600 Elderberries
4,450 Peppers, sweet red	600 Green beans
4,300 Hubbard squash	590 Watermelon
3,400 Cantaloupe	580 Rutabagas
3,300 Butter	550 Brussels sprouts
3,300 Endive	520 Okra
2,700 Apricots	510 Yellow cornmeal
2,500 Broccoli spears	460 Yellow squash
2,260 Whitefish	

Vitamin A from animal sources occurs mostly as active, pre-formed Vitamin A (retinol), while that from vegetable sources occurs as provitamin A (beta-carotene and other carotenoids) which must be converted to active Vitamin A by the body to be utilized. The efficiency of conversion varies among individuals; however, beta-carotene is converted more efficiently than other carotenoids. Green and deep yellow vegetables as well as deep yellow fruits are highest in beta-carotene.

Vitamin B Complex

B1 Thiamin

Milligrams (mg) per 100 grams edible portion
(100 grams = 3 1/2 ounces)

15.61 Brewer's yeast	0.45 Heart, lamb
14.01 Torula yeast	0.45 Wild rice
2.01 Wheat germ	0.43 Cashews
1.96 Sunflower seeds	0.43 Rye, whole-grain
1.28 Pine nuts	0.40 Lobster
1.14 Peanuts, with skins	0.38 Cornmeal, whole-ground
1.10 Soybeans, dry	0.38 Mung beans
0.98 Peanuts, without skins	0.37 Lentils
0.96 Brazil nuts	0.35 Green peas
0.86 Pecans	0.34 Brown rice
0.85 Soybean flour	0.34 Macadamia nuts
0.74 Split peas	0.33 Walnuts
0.73 Millet	0.31 Garbanzos
0.72 Wheat bran	0.25 Garlic cloves
0.67 Pistachio nuts	0.24 Almonds
0.65 Navy beans	0.24 Lima beans, fresh
0.64 Beans, pinto and red	0.24 Pumpkin and squash seeds
0.63 Heart, veal	0.23 Chestnuts, fresh
0.60 Buckwheat	0.23 Soybean sprouts
0.60 Oatmeal	0.22 Peppers, red chili
0.55 Whole wheat flour	0.18 Sesame seeds, hulled
0.55 Whole wheat	
0.48 Lima beans, dry	
0.46 Hazelnuts	

B2 Riboflavin

Milligrams (mg) per 100 grams edible portion
(100 grams = 3 1/2 ounces)

5.06 Torula yeast	0.25 Rice bran
4.28 Brewer's yeast	0.25 Veal
0.92 Almonds	0.24 Lamb, lean
0.68 Wheat germ	0.23 Broccoli
0.63 Wild rice	0.23 Chicken, flesh and skin
0.46 Mushrooms	0.23 Pine nuts
0.44 Egg yolks	0.23 Salmon
0.38 Millet	0.23 Sunflower seeds
0.36 Peppers, hot red	0.22 Beet and mustard
0.35 Soy flour	greens
0.35 Wheat bran	0.22 Lentils
0.33 Mackerel	0.22 Navy beans
0.31 Collard greens	0.22 Prunes
0.31 Eggs	0.22 Rye, whole grain
0.31 Soybeans, dry	0.21 Beans, pinto and red
0.29 Split peas	0.21 Mung beans
0.26 Kale	0.21 Black-eyed peas
0.26 Parsley	0.21 Okra
0.25 Cashews	0.13 Sesame seeds, hulled

B3 Niacin

Milligrams (mg) per 100 grams edible portion
(100 grams = 3 1/2 ounces)

44.4 Torula yeast	10.7 Chicken, light meat
37.9 Brewer's yeast	8.4 Trout
29.8 Rice bran	8.3 Halibut
21.0 Wheat bran	8.2 Mackerel
17.2 Peanuts, with skins	8.0 Chicken, flesh only
15.8 Peanuts, without skins	8.0 Turkey, flesh only
11.3 Turkey, light meat	7.2 Salmon

6.4 Veal
6.2 Wild rice
5.7 Lamb, lean
5.6 Chicken, flesh and skin
5.4 Sesame seeds
5.4 Sunflower seeds
5.1 Beef, lean
4.7 Brown rice
4.5 Pine nuts
4.4 Buckwheat, whole-grain
4.4 Peppers, red chili

4.4 Whole wheat grain
4.3 Whole wheat flour
4.2 Mushrooms
4.2 Wheat germ
3.7 Barley
3.6 Herring
3.5 Almonds
3.2 Shrimp
3.0 Haddock
3.0 Split peas

B5 Pantothenic Acid

Milligrams (mg) per 100 grams edible portion
(100 grams = 3 1/2 ounces)

12.0 Brewer's yeast
11.0 Torula yeast
2.8 Peanuts
2.2 Mushrooms
2.0 Soybean flour
2.0 Split peas
1.9 Perch
1.8 Blue cheese
1.7 Pecans
1.7 Soybeans
1.6 Eggs
1.5 Lobster
1.5 Oatmeal, dry
1.4 Buckwheat flour
1.4 Lentils
1.4 Sunflower seeds
1.3 Cashews
1.3 Rye flour, whole

1.3 Salmon, flesh
1.2 Camembert cheese
1.2 Garbanzos
1.2 Wheat germ, toasted
1.2 Broccoli
1.1 Brown rice
1.1 Avocados
1.1 Hazelnuts
1.1 Wheat flour, whole
1.1 Peppers, red chilli
1.1 Sardines
1.1 Veal, lean
1.1 Turkey, dark meat
1.0 Black-eyed peas, dry
1.0 Cauliflower
1.0 Chicken, dark meat
1.0 Kale
1.0 Wild rice

B6 Pyridoxine

Milligrams (mg) per 100 grams edible portion
(100 grams = 3 1/2 ounces)

3.00 Torula yeast	0.34 Whole wheat flour
2.50 Brewer's yeast	0.33 Chestnuts, fresh
1.25 Sunflower seeds	0.30 Egg yolks
1.15 Wheat germ, toasted	0.30 Kale
0.90 Tuna, flesh	0.30 Rye flour
0.81 Soybeans, dry	0.26 Turnip greens
0.73 Walnuts	0.26 Peppers, sweet
0.70 Salmon, flesh	0.28 Spinach
0.69 Trout, flesh	0.25 Potatoes
0.66 Mackerel, flesh	0.24 Prunes
0.63 Soybean flour	0.24 Raisins
0.60 Lentils, dry	0.24 Sardines
0.58 Buckwheat flour	0.23 Brussels sprouts
0.58 Lima beans, dry	0.23 Elderberries
0.56 Black-eyed peas, dry	0.23 Perch, flesh
0.56 Navy beans, dry	0.22 Barley
0.55 Brown rice	0.22 Cheese, Camembert
0.54 Garbanzos, dry	0.22 Cod, flesh
0.54 Hazelnuts	0.22 Sweet potatoes
0.53 Pinto beans, dry	0.21 Cauliflower
0.51 Bananas	0.20 Leeks
0.44 Albacore, flesh	0.20 Molasses
0.43 Beef, lean	0.20 Popcorn, popped
0.43 Halibut, flesh	0.20 Red cabbage
0.42 Avocados	

B7 Biotin

Micrograms (mcg) per 100 grams edible portion
(100 grams = 3 1/2 ounces)

200 Brewer's yeast	24 Sardines, canned
70 Soy flour	22 Whole egg
61 Soybeans	21 Black-eyed peas
60 Rice bran	18 Almonds
58 Rice germ	18 Split peas
57 Rice polishings	17 Cauliflower
52 Egg yolk	16 Mushrooms
39 Peanut butter	16 Whole wheat cereal
37 Walnuts	15 Salmon, canned
34 Peanuts, roasted	14 Bran
31 Barley	13 Lentils
27 Pecans	12 Brown rice
24 Oatmeal	10 Chicken

B9 Folic Acid

Micrograms (mcg) per 100 grams edible portion
(100 grams = 3 1/2 ounces)

2,022 Brewer's yeast	105 Lentils
440 Black-eyed peas	77 Walnuts
430 Rice germ	75 Spinach, fresh
425 Soy flour	70 Kale
305 Wheat germ	65 Filbert nuts
225 Soybeans	60 Beet greens and mustard greens
195 Bran	56 Peanut butter
180 Kidney beans	56 Peanuts, roasted
145 Mung beans	53 Broccoli
130 Lima beans	50 Barley
125 Navy beans	50 Split peas
125 Garbanzos	49 Brussels sprouts
110 Asparagus	

45 Almonds
38 Whole wheat flour
33 Oatmeal
32 Cabbage
32 Figs, dried
30 Avocado
28 Coconut, fresh
28 Green beans

28 Corn
27 Pecans
25 Dates
25 Mushrooms
14 Blackberries
7 Ground beef
5 Orange

B10 Para-aminobenzoic Acid (PABA)

As food sources with appreciable quantities of this nutrient are few, a listing of the best sources of this nutrient is given instead of showing relative nutrient amounts

Bran
Cabbage
Eggs
Mushrooms
Oats

Spinach
Sunflower Seeds
Wheat Germ
Whole Milk

B12 Cyanocobalamin

Micrograms (mcg) per 100 grams edible portion
(100 grams = 3 1/2 ounces)

98 Clams
18 Oysters
17 Sardines
6.0 Egg yolks
5.0 Trout
4.0 Salmon, flesh
3.0 Tuna, flesh
2.1 Lamb
2.0 Eggs
2.0 Whey, dried
1.8 Beef, lean
1.8 Edam cheese

1.8 Swiss cheese
1.6 Brie cheese
1.6 Gruyere cheese
1.4 Blue cheese
1.3 Haddock, flesh
1.2 Flounder, flesh
1.2 Scallops
1.0 Cheddar cheese
1.0 Cottage cheese
1.0 Mozzarella cheese
1.0 Halibut
1.0 Perch, fillets

B15 Pangamic Acid

As food sources with appreciable quantities of this nutrient are few, a listing of the best sources of this nutrient is given instead of showing relative nutrient amounts

Apricot kernels	Sunflower seeds
Corn grits	Wheat bran
Oat grits	Wheat germ
Pumpkin seeds	Whole grain cereals
Rice bran	Yeast

Vitamin B17 Amygdalin (sometimes called laetrile)

HIGH: Above 500 milligrams (mg) per 100 grams edible portion

Alfalfa leaves	Macadamia nuts
Apple seeds	Mung beans
Apricot seeds	Nectarine seeds
Bamboo sprouts	Peach seed
Bitter almond	Pear seed
Cherry seeds	Plum seed
Elderberry	Prune seed
Fava beans	Wild blackberry

MEDIUM: Above 100 milligrams (mg) per 100 grams edible portion

Alfalfa sprouts	Lentils
Black-eyed peas	Lima beans
Boysenberry	Loganberry
Buckwheat	Millet
Currant	Mulberry
Flaxseed	Mung bean sprouts
Garbanzo beans	Quince
Gooseberry	Raspberry
Huckleberry	Squash seed
Kidney beans	

LOW: Below 100 milligrams (mg) per 100 grams edible portion

Beet tops	Green peas
Black beans	Lima beans
Cashews	Spinach
Commercial blackberry	Sweet potatoes, yams
Cranberry	Watercress

Choline

Micrograms (mcg) per 100 grams edible portion
(100 grams = 3 1/2 ounces)

2,200 Lecithin	139 Barley
1,490 Egg yolk	112 Brown rice
504 Whole egg	104 Veal
406 Wheat germ	86 Molasses
340 Soybeans	75 Beef
300 Rice germ	75 Green peas
257 Black-eyed peas	66 Sweet potatoes
245 Garbanzo beans	48 Cheddar cheese
240 Brewer's yeast	42 Green beans
223 Lentils	29 Potatoes
201 Split peas	23 Cabbage
170 Rice bran	22 Spinach
162 Peanuts, roasted	15 Milk
156 Oatmeal	12 Orange juice
145 Peanut butter	5 Butter
143 Bran	

Inositol

Milligrams (mg) per 100 grams edible portion
(100 grams = 3 1/2 ounces)

2,200 Lecithin	500 Navy beans
770 Wheat germ	460 Rice bran

390 Cooked barley
370 Rice germ
370 Whole wheat
270 Oatmeal
270 Brewer's yeast
240 Garbanzo beans
240 Black-eyed peas
210 Orange
205 Soy flour
200 Soybeans
180 Peanuts, roasted
180 Peanut butter
170 Lima beans
162 Green peas
150 Grapefruit
150 Molasses
150 Split peas
130 Lentils

120 Cantaloupe
120 Raisins
119 Brown rice
117 Orange juice
110 Whole wheat flour
96 Peaches
95 Cabbage
95 Cauliflower
88 Onion
67 Whole wheat bread
66 Sweet potatoes
64 Watermelon
60 Strawberries
55 Lettuce
46 Tomato
33 Egg
13 Milk
11 Beef, round

Vitamin C Ascorbic Acid

Milligrams (mg) per 100 grams edible portion
(100 grams = 3 1/2 ounces)

1,300 Acerola
369 Peppers, red chili
242 Guavas
204 Peppers, red sweet
186 Kale leaves
172 Parsley
152 Collard greens
139 Turnip greens
128 Peppers, green sweet
113 Broccoli
102 Brussels sprouts
97 Mustard greens

79 Watercress
78 Cauliflower
66 Persimmons
61 Cabbage, red
59 Strawberries
56 Papayas
51 Spinach
50 Oranges and juice
41 Cabbage
46 Lemon juice
38 Grapefruits and juice
36 Elderberries

36 Turnips

35 Mangos

33 Asparagus

33 Cantaloupes

32 Green onions

32 Swiss chard

31 Okra

31 Tangerines

30 Oysters

29 Black-eyed peas

29 Lima beans, young

29 Soybeans

27 Green peas

26 Radishes

25 Chinese cabbage

25 Raspberries

25 Yellow summer squash

24 Loganberries

23 Honeydew melon

23 Tomatoes

Bioflavonoids

As food sources with appreciable quantities of this nutrient are few, a listing of the best sources of this nutrient is given instead of showing relative nutrient amounts

Apricots	Lemon juice
Black currant	Orange
Blackberry	Papaya
Broccoli	Parsley
Cabbage	Peppers
Cantaloupe	Plums
Cherries	Prunes
Grapefruit	Rose hips
Grapes	Tomato

Vitamin D

IU per 100 grams edible portion (100 grams = 3 1/2 ounces)

500 Sardines, canned	90 Sunflower seeds
350 Salmon	50 Eggs
250 Tuna	40 Milk, fortified
150 Shrimp	40 Mushrooms
90 Butter	30 Natural cheeses

Vitamin E

IU per 100 grams edible portion (100 grams = 3 1/2 ounces)

216 Wheat germ oil	3.0 Bran
90 Sunflower seeds	2.9 Asparagus
88 Sunflower seed oil	2.5 Brown rice
72 Safflower oil	2.5 Salmon
48 Almonds	2.3 Rye, whole
45 Sesame oil	2.2 Rye bread, dark
34 Peanut oil	1.9 Pecans
29 Corn oil	1.9 Rye and wheat crackers
22 Wheat germ	1.9 Wheat germ
16 Peanuts	1.4 Whole wheat bread
18 Olive oil	1.0 Carrots
14 Soybean oil	0.99 Peas
13 Peanuts, roasted	0.92 Walnuts
11 Peanut butter	0.88 Bananas
3.6 Butter	0.83 Eggs
3.2 Spinach	0.72 Tomatoes
3.0 Oatmeal	0.29 Lamb

Vitamin K

Micrograms (mcg) per 100 grams edible portion
(100 grams = 3 1/2 ounces)

650 Turnip greens	19 Green peas
200 Broccoli	17 Whole wheat
129 Lettuce	14 Green beans
125 Cabbage	11 Eggs
89 Spinach	8 Peaches
57 Watercress	7 Beef
57 Asparagus	6 Raisins
35 Cheese	5 Tomato
30 Butter	3 Milk
20 Oats	3 Potato

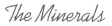
The Minerals

Calcium

Milligrams (mg) per 100 grams edible portion
(100 grams = 3 1/2 ounces)

1,093 Kelp	103 Broccoli
925 Swiss cheese	99 English walnut
750 Cheddar cheese	94 Cottage cheese
352 Carob flour	93 Spinach
296 Dulse	73 Pecans
250 Collard greens	73 Soybeans, cooked
246 Turnip greens	72 Wheat germ
245 Barbados molasses	69 Peanuts
234 Almonds	68 Miso
213 Kale	68 Romaine lettuce
210 Brewer's yeast	67 Dried apricots
203 Parsley	66 Rutabaga
200 Corn tortillas (lime added)	62 Raisins
187 Dandelion greens	60 Black currant
186 Brazil nuts	59 Carrot juice
151 Watercress	59 Dates
129 Goat milk	56 Green snap beans
128 Tofu	51 Globe artichoke
126 Figs, dried	51 Prunes, dried
121 Buttermilk	51 Pumpkin and squash seeds
120 Sunflower seeds	50 Cooked dry beans
120 Yogurt	49 Common cabbage
119 Beet greens	48 Soybean sprouts
119 Wheat bran	46 Hard winter wheat
118 Whole milk	41 Orange
114 Buckwheat, raw	39 Celery
110 Sesame seeds, hulled	38 Cashews
106 Ripe olives	38 Rye grain

37 Carrot	19 Mung bean sprouts
34 Barley	17 Pineapple
32 Brown rice	16 Beets
32 Sweet potato	16 Grapes
29 Garlic	14 Cantaloupe
28 Summer squash	14 Jerusalem artichoke
27 Onion	13 Tomato
26 Fresh green peas	12 Chicken
26 Lemon	12 Eggplant
25 Cauliflower	11 Orange juice
25 Lentils, cooked	10 Avocado
22 Asparagus	10 Beef
22 Sweet cherry	8 Banana
22 Winter squash	7 Apple
21 Strawberry	3 Sweet corn
20 Millet	

Chromium

Micrograms (mcg) per 100 grams edible portion
(100 grams = 3 1/2 ounces)

112 Brewer's yeast*	13 Butter
57 Beef, round	13 Parsnips
42 Whole wheat bread*	12 Cornmeal
38 Wheat bran	12 Lamb chop
30 Rye bread	11 Scallops
30 Fresh chili	11 Swiss cheese
26 Oysters	10 Banana
24 Potatoes	10 Spinach
23 Wheat germ	9 Carrots
19 Green pepper	8 Navy beans, dry
16 Eggs	7 Lettuce
15 Chicken	7 Shrimp
14 Apple	5 Blueberries

5 Lobster tail   4 Mushrooms
5 Orange   3 Beer
4 Cabbage   3 Strawberries
4 Green beans   1 Milk

NOTE: The above values show total chromium content of these foods and do not indicate the amount that may biologically be active as the Glucose Tolerance Factor (GTF). Those foods marked with an asterisk are high in GTF.

Copper

Milligrams (mg) per 100 grams edible portion
(100 grams = 3 1/2 ounces)

3.7 Oysters	0.3 Carrot
2.3 Brazil nuts	0.3 Clams
2.1 Soy lecithin	0.3 Coconut
1.4 Almonds	0.3 Garlic
1.3 Hazelnuts	0.3 Olive oil
1.3 Walnuts	0.3 Shrimp
1.3 Pecans	0.2 Chicken
1.2 Split peas, dry	0.2 Corn oil
0.8 Buckwheat	0.2 Eggs
0.8 Peanuts	0.2 Gingerroot
0.7 Cod liver oil	0.2 Millet
0.7 Lamb chops	0.2 Molasses
0.5 Sunflower oil	0.2 Whole wheat
0.4 Barley	0.2 Turnips
0.4 Butter	0.1 Apple
0.4 Gelatin	0.1 Green peas
0.4 Rye grain	0.1 Papaya

Black pepper, thyme, paprika, bay leaves, and active dry yeast are also high in copper.

Iodine

Micrograms (mcg) per 100 grams edible portion
(100 grams = 3 1/2 ounces)

90 Clams	11 Whole wheat bread
65 Shrimp	10 Lettuce
62 Haddock	9 Butter
50 Oysters	9 Green peppers
50 Salmon	9 Spinach
46 Halibut	7 Milk
37 Sardines, canned	6 Beef
16 Pineapple	6 Cottage cheese
16 Tuna, canned	6 Cream
14 Eggs	3 Lamb
11 Cheddar cheese	3 Raisins
11 Peanuts	

Iron

Milligrams (mg) per 100 grams edible portion
(100 grams = 3 1/2 ounces)

100.0 Kelp	3.7 Lean beef
17.3 Brewer's yeast	3.5 Raisins
16.1 Blackstrap molasses	3.4 Brazil nuts
14.9 Wheat bran	3.4 Jerusalem artichoke
11.2 Pumpkin and squash seeds	3.3 Beet greens
9.4 Wheat germ	3.2 Swiss chard
7.1 Sunflower seeds	3.1 Dandelion greens
6.8 Millet	3.1 English walnut
6.2 Parsley	3.0 Dates
6.1 Clams	2.7 Cooked dry beans
4.7 Almonds	2.4 Sesame seeds, hulled
3.9 Prunes, dried	2.4 Pecans
3.8 Cashews	2.3 Eggs
	2.1 Lentils

2.1 Peanuts
1.9 Lamb
1.9 Tofu
1.8 Green peas
1.6 Brown rice
1.6 Ripe olives
1.5 Chicken
1.3 Artichoke
1.3 Mung bean sprouts
1.2 Salmon
1.1 Broccoli
1.1 Cauliflower
1.1 Currants
1.1 Whole wheat bread
1.0 Asparagus
1.0 Cheddar cheese
1.0 Strawberry
0.9 Blackberries
0.8 Red cabbage
0.8 Pumpkin
0.8 Mushrooms
0.7 Banana

0.7 Beets
0.7 Carrot
0.7 Eggplant
0.7 Sweet potato
0.6 Avocado
0.6 Corn
0.6 Figs
0.6 Potato
0.5 Pineapple
0.5 Nectarine
0.5 Watermelon
0.5 Winter squash
0.5 Brown rice, cooked
0.5 Tomato
0.4 Orange
0.4 Cherries
0.4 Summer squash
0.3 Papaya
0.3 Celery
0.3 Cottage cheese
0.3 Apple

Magnesium

Milligrams (mg) per 100 grams edible portion
(100 grams = 3 1/2 ounces)

760 Kelp
490 Wheat bran, cooked
336 Wheat germ
270 Almonds
267 Cashews
258 Blackstrap molasses
231 Brewer's yeast
229 Buckwheat

225 Brazil nut
220 Dulse
184 Filberts
175 Peanuts
162 Millet
160 Wheat grain, whole
142 Pecan
131 English walnut

115 Rye
111 Tofu
106 Beet greens
90 Coconut meat, dry
88 Brown rice
88 Soybeans, cooked
88 Spinach
71 Eggs, dried
65 Swiss chard
62 Apricots, dried
58 Dates
57 Collard greens
51 Shrimp
48 Sweet corn
45 Avocado
45 Cheddar cheese
41 Parsley
40 Prunes, dried
38 Sunflower seeds
37 Barley
37 Common beans, cooked
36 Dandelion greens
36 Garlic
35 Raisins
35 Fresh green peas
34 Crab
34 Potato with skin

33 Banana
31 Sweet potato
30 Blackberry
25 Beets
24 Broccoli
24 Cauliflower
23 Carrot
22 Celery
21 Beef
20 Asparagus
19 Chicken
18 Green pepper
17 Winter squash
16 Cantaloupe
16 Eggplant
14 Tomato
13 Cabbage
13 Grapes
13 Milk
13 Mushroom
13 Pineapple
12 Onion
11 Orange
11 Iceberg lettuce
9 Plum
8 Apple

Manganese

Milligrams (mg) per 100 grams edible portion
(100 grams = 3 1/2 ounces)

3.5 Pecans
2.8 Brazil nuts
2.5 Almonds

1.8 Barley
1.3 Buckwheat
1.3 Rye

1.3 Split peas, dry
1.1 Whole wheat
0.8 Fresh spinach
0.8 Walnuts
0.6 Oats
0.5 Raisins
0.5 Rhubarb
0.5 Turnip greens
0.4 Beet greens
0.3 Brussels sprouts
0.3 Oatmeal
0.2 Cornmeal
0.2 Millet
0.19 Gorgonzola cheese
0.16 Carrots
0.15 Broccoli
0.14 Brown rice
0.14 Whole wheat bread
0.13 Corn
0.13 Swiss cheese
0.11 Cabbage

0.10 Peach
0.10 Peanuts
0.09 Butter
0.06 Peas
0.06 Tangerine
0.05 Eggs
0.04 Beets
0.04 Coconut
0.03 Apple
0.03 Cantaloupe
0.03 Lamb chops
0.03 Orange
0.03 Pear
0.03 Tomato
0.02 Apricot
0.02 Chicken breasts
0.02 Green beans
0.02 Whole milk
0.01 Cucumber
0.01 Halibut
0.01 Scallops

Clover, ginger, thyme, bay leaves, and tea are also high in manganese.

Molybdenum

Micrograms (mcg) per 100 grams edible portion
(100 grams = 3 1/2 ounces)

155 Lentils
130 Split peas
120 Cauliflower
110 Green peas
109 Brewer's yeast
100 Spinach

100 Wheat germ
75 Brown rice
70 Garlic
60 Oats
53 Eggs
50 Rye bread

45 Corn
42 Barley
40 Fish
36 Whole wheat grain
32 Chicken
32 Whole wheat bread
31 Cottage cheese
30 Beef
30 Potatoes
25 Coconut
25 Onions
25 Peanuts
24 Lamb

21 Green beans
19 Crab
19 Molasses
16 Cantaloupe
14 Apricots
10 Butter
10 Raisins
7 Strawberries
5 Cabbage
5 Carrots
3 Whole milk
1 Goat milk

Nickel

Micrograms (mcg) per 100 grams edible portion
(100 grams = 3 1/2 ounces)

700 Soybeans, dry
500 Beans, dry
410 Soy flour
310 Lentils
250 Split peas
175 Green peas
153 Green beans
150 Oats
132 Walnuts
122 Hazelnuts
100 Buckwheat
90 Barley
90 Corn
90 Parsley
36 Whole wheat
35 Spinach
30 Fish

27 Cucumber
25 Carrots
25 Rye bread
24 Eggs
22 Cabbage
20 Onions
20 Tomatoes
16 Apricots
16 Beef
16 Oranges
16 Potatoes
15 Cheese
15 Watermelon
14 Lettuce
13 Apples
12 Whole wheat bread
12 Beets

12 Pears
8 Grapes
6 Lamb

6 Pine nuts
6 Radishes
3 Milk

Phosphorus

Milligrams (mg) per 100 grams edible portion
(100 grams = 3 1/2 ounces)

1,753 Brewer's yeast
1,276 Wheat bran
1,144 Pumpkin and squash seeds
1,118 Wheat germ
837 Sunflower seeds
693 Brazil nuts
592 Sesame seeds, hulled
554 Soybeans, dried
504 Almonds
478 Cheddar cheese
457 Pinto beans, dried
409 Peanuts
400 Wheat
380 English walnuts
376 Rye grain
373 Cashews
338 Scallops
311 Millet
290 Barley, pearled
289 Pecans
267 Dulse
240 Kelp
239 Chicken
221 Brown rice
205 Eggs
202 Garlic

175 Crab
152 Cottage cheese
150 Beef or lamb
119 Lentils, cooked
116 Fresh peas
116 Mushrooms
111 Sweet corn
101 Raisins
93 Whole cow's milk
88 Globe artichoke
87 Yogurt
80 Brussels sprouts
79 Prunes, dried
78 Broccoli
77 Figs, dried
69 Yams
67 Soybean sprouts
64 Mung bean sprouts
63 Dates
63 Parsley
62 Asparagus
59 Bamboo shoots
56 Cauliflower
53 Potato with skin
51 Okra
51 Spinach
44 Green beans

44 Pumpkin
42 Avocado
40 Beet greens
39 Swiss chard
38 Winter squash
36 Carrot
36 Onions
35 Red cabbage
33 Beets
31 Radish
29 Summer squash
28 Celery
27 Cucumber

27 Tomato
26 Banana
26 Eggplant
26 Lettuce
26 Persimmon
24 Nectarine
22 Raspberry
20 Grapes
20 Orange
17 Olives
16 Cantaloupe
10 Apple
8 Pineapple

Potassium

Milligrams (mg) per 100 grams edible portion
(100 grams = 3 1/2 ounces)

8,060 Dulse
5,273 Kelp
920 Sunflower seeds
827 Wheat germ
773 Almonds
763 Raisins
727 Parsley
715 Brazil nuts
674 Peanuts
648 Dates
640 Figs, dried
604 Avocado
603 Pecans
600 Yams
550 Swiss chard
540 Soybeans, cooked
529 Garlic

470 Spinach
450 English walnuts
430 Millet
416 Beans, cooked
414 Mushrooms
407 Potato with skin
382 Broccoli
370 Banana
370 Meats
369 Winter squash
366 Chicken
341 Carrots
341 Celery
322 Radishes
295 Cauliflower
282 Watercress
278 Asparagus

268 Red cabbage
264 Lettuce
251 Cantaloupe
249 Lentils, cooked
244 Tomato
243 Sweet potato
234 Papaya
214 Eggplant
213 Green pepper
208 Beets
202 Peach
202 Summer squash
200 Orange
199 Raspberries

191 Cherries
164 Strawberry
162 Grapefruit juice
158 Grapes
157 Onions
146 Pineapple
144 Milk, whole
141 Lemon juice
130 Pear
129 Eggs
110 Apple
100 Watermelon
70 Brown rice, cooked

Selenium

Micrograms (mcg) per 100 grams edible portion
(100 grams = 3 1/2 ounces)

146 Butter
141 Smoked herring
123 Smelt
111 Wheat germ
103 Brazil nuts
89 Apple cider vinegar
77 Scallops
66 Barley
66 Whole wheat bread
65 Lobster
63 Bran
59 Shrimp
57 Red swiss chard
56 Oats
55 Clams
51 King crab

49 Oysters
48 Milk
43 Cod
39 Brown rice
34 Top round steak
30 Lamb
27 Turnips
26 Molasses
25 Garlic
19 Gelatin
19 Orange juice
18 Egg yolk
18 Lamb chop
12 Chicken
12 Mushrooms
10 Swiss cheese

5 Cottage cheese
4 Grape juice
4 Radishes
3 Pecans
2 Almonds
2 Cabbage

2 Carrots
2 Green beans
2 Hazelnuts
2 Kidney beans
2 Onion
1 Orange

Sodium

Milligrams (mg) per 100 grams edible portion
(100 grams = 3 1/2 ounces)

3,007 Kelp	47 Carrot
2,400 Green olives	47 Yogurt
1,428 Dill pickles	45 Parsley
828 Ripe olives	43 Artichoke
747 Sauerkraut	34 Figs, dried
700 Cheddar cheese	30 Lentils, dried
265 Scallops	30 Sunflower seeds
229 Cottage cheese	27 Raisins
210 Lobster	26 Red cabbage
147 Swiss chard	19 Garlic
130 Beet greens	19 White beans
130 Buttermilk	15 Broccoli
126 Celery	15 Mushrooms
122 Eggs	13 Cauliflower
110 Cod	10 Onion
71 Spinach	10 Sweet potato
70 Lamb	9 Brown rice
64 Chicken	9 Lettuce
60 Beef	6 Cucumber
60 Beets	5 Peanuts
60 Sesame seeds	4 Avocado
52 Watercress	3 Tomato
50 Whole cow's milk	2 Eggplant
49 Turnip	

2,132 Salt, 1 teaspoon
1,319 Soy sauce, 1 tablespoon

The following foods contain large amounts of sodium chloride added during processing and should generally be avoided:

Canned or frozen vegetables	Potato chips, corn chips, pretzels, etc.
Cured, smoked, or canned meats	Luncheon meats
Packaged spice mixes	Salted nuts
Bouillon cubes	Salted crackers
Canned fish	Canned or packaged soups
Commercial peanut butter	Processed cheeses
Ketchup, barbecue sauce	Commercial salad dressings
	Meat tenderizers

Vanadium

Micrograms (mcg) per 100 grams edible portion
(100 grams = 3 1/2 ounces)

100 Buckwheat	10 Garlic
80 Parsley	6 Tomatoes
70 Soybeans	5 Onions
42 Eggs	5 Radishes
35 Oats	5 Whole wheat
30 Olive oil	4 Beets
15 Corn	4 Lobster
15 Sunflower seeds	3 Apples
14 Green beans	2 Lettuce
11 Peanut oil	2 Millet
10 Carrots	2 Plums
10 Cabbage	

Zinc

Milligrams (mg) per 100 grams edible portion
(100 grams = 3 1/2 ounces)

148.7 Fresh oysters	1.6 Green peas
6.8 Gingerroot	1.5 Shrimp
5.6 Ground round steak	1.2 Turnips
5.3 Lamb chops	0.9 Parsley
4.5 Pecans	0.9 Potatoes
4.2 Brazil nuts	0.6 Garlic
4.2 Split peas, dry	0.5 Carrots
3.5 Nonfat dry milk	0.5 Whole wheat bread
3.5 Egg yolk	0.4 Black beans
3.2 Oats	0.4 Corn
3.2 Peanuts	0.4 Pork chop
3.2 Rye	0.4 Raw milk
3.2 Whole wheat	0.3 Grape juice
3.1 Almonds	0.3 Olive oil
3.1 Lima beans	0.3 Cauliflower
3.1 Soy lecithin	0.2 Butter
3.0 Walnuts	0.2 Cabbage
2.9 Sardines	0.2 Lentils
2.6 Chicken	0.2 Lettuce
2.5 Buckwheat	0.2 Spinach
2.4 Hazelnuts	0.1 Cucumber
1.9 Clams	0.1 String beans
1.7 Anchovies	0.1 Tangerine
1.7 Haddock	0.1 Yams
1.7 Tuna	

Black pepper, paprika, mustard, chili powder, thyme, and cinnamon are also high in zinc.

CHAPTER TEN

Recipes for Fasting and Detoxing

Most of the recipes here use vegetables, herbs, nuts, and seeds, and nut or seed milk for the smoothies. A few recipes have half of a low-sugar apple or pear for flavor. It's a healthful choice to avoid fruit juice as much as possible, since it contains too much fruit sugar and some can be acidic. The goal in the detox programs and maintenance diet is to alkalinize your body. When you do choose to add a little fruit for flavor, make sure it is low in sugar and always diluted with lots of vegetable juice.

Low-Sugar Fruit	
Lemons	Berries
Limes	Green Apples
Grapefruit	Pears

Vegetable Juice Recipes

MORNING ENERGY

3 to 4 carrots, scrubbed
  well, tops removed,
  ends trimmed
1 cucumber, peeled
1/2 beet, scrubbed well
  (may include stem and
  1 or 2 leaves)

1/2 lemon, peeled
1-inch chunk gingerroot,
  scrubbed, or peeled
  if old

Cut produce to fit your juicer's feed tube. Juice all ingredients
and stir. Pour into a glass and drink as soon as possible.
SERVES 1 TO 2

BEET-CUCUMBER CLEANSING COCKTAIL

1 cucumber, peeled
3 carrots, scrubbed well,
  tops removed, ends
  trimmed
1 beet, scrubbed well, with
  stem and 1 or 2 leaves
2 stalks celery

1 handful parsley
1- to 2-inch chunk gingerroot, scrubbed, or
  peeled if old
1/2 lemon, peeled

Cut produce to fit your juicer's feed tube. Juice all ingredients
and stir. Pour into a glass and drink as soon as possible.
SERVES 1 TO 2

SPRING CLEANSING COCKTAIL

1 vine-ripened tomato   *8 asparagus stalks*
1 cucumber, peeled   *1/2 lemon, peeled*

Cut produce to fit your juicer's feed tube. Juice all ingredients and stir. Pour into a glass and drink as soon as possible.
SERVES 1 TO 2

Note: Asparagus is a natural diuretic, which helps flush toxins from the body and promotes kidney cleansing.

LIVER-CLEANSING COCKTAIL

1 handful dandelion   *1/2 cucumber, peeled*
greens   *1/2 lemon, peeled*
3 to 4 carrots, scrubbed
well, tops removed,
ends trimmed

Bunch up dandelion greens. Cut produce to fit your juicer's feed tube. Tuck the greens in feed tube and push through with a carrot. Juice remaining ingredients, finishing with a carrot. Stir the juice, pour into a glass, and drink as soon as possible.
SERVES 1

Note: Dandelion juice is a traditional remedy for cleansing the liver.

CUCUMBER REFRESHER

1 cucumber, peeled   *1/2 lemon, peeled*

Cut produce to fit your juicer's feed tube. Juice ingredients and stir. Pour into a glass and drink as soon as possible.
SERVES 1

DIANE'S DELIGHT

1 cucumber, peeled
2 to 3 stalks celery, leaves can be included
1/2 lemon, with peel, seeded (use only organic)

1-inch chunk gingerroot, scrubbed, or peeled if old

Cut produce to fit your juicer's feed tube. Juice ingredients and stir. Pour into a glass and drink as soon as possible.
SERVES 1 TO 2

THE ORIENT EXPRESS

2-inch by 4- or 5-inch chunk of jicama, scrubbed well or peeled
2 to 3 carrots, scrubbed well, tops removed, ends trimmed

1 daikon radish, trimmed and scrubbed
1-inch chunk gingerroot, scrubbed, or peeled if old

Cut produce to fit your juicer's feed tube. Juice ingredients and stir. Pour into a glass and drink as soon as possible.
SERVES 1

SALSA IN A GLASS

1 medium vine-ripened
    tomato
1/2 cucumber, peeled
1 small handful cilantro

1/2 lime, peeled
Dash of hot sauce
    (optional)

Cut produce to fit your juicer's feed tube. Juice ingredients
and stir. Pour into a glass and drink as soon as possible.
SERVES 1

SPICY TOMATO

2 medium vine-ripened
    tomatoes
2 dark green lettuce leaves

2 radishes, scrubbed
4 sprigs parsley
1/2 lime or lemon, peeled

Cut produce to fit your juicer's feed tube. Juice ingredients
and stir. Pour into a glass and drink as soon as possible.
SERVES 1

TOMATO FLORENTINE

2 vine-ripened tomatoes
1 large handful spinach

4 to 5 sprigs basil
1/2 lemon, peeled

Juice one tomato. Wrap the basil in several spinach leaves.
Turn off the machine and add the spinach and basil. Turn
the machine back on and gently tap to juice them. Juice the
remaining tomato and lemon. Stir juice, pour in a glass,
and drink as soon as possible.
SERVES 1

CABBAGE COCKTAIL

1/4 small head green
   cabbage
3 carrots, scrubbed well,
   tops removed, ends
   trimmed

4 celery stalks, with leaves
   if desired

Cut produce to fit your juicer's feed tube. Juice ingredients and stir. Pour into a glass and drink as soon as possible.
SERVES 1

SPINACH POWER

1/2 cucumber, peeled
3 carrots, scrubbed well,
   tops removed, ends
   trimmed
2 celery stalks, with leaves
   as desired

1/2 beet, scrubbed well
   (may include stem and
   1 to 2 leaves)
1 small handful parsley
1/2 lemon, peeled

Cut produce to fit your juicer's feed tube. Juice ingredients and stir. Pour into a glass and drink as soon as possible.
SERVES 1 TO 2

SUPER GREEN DRINK

1 cucumber, peeled
1 large handful spinach
1 large handful sunflower
   sprouts

1 small handful
   buckwheat sprouts
1 small handful clover
   sprouts

Cut the cucumber to fit your juicer's feed tube. Juice part of the cucumber first. Bunch up the sprouts and wrap in spinach leaves, turn off the machine and add them. Turn the machine back on and tap with the rest of the cucumber to gently push the sprouts and spinach through, and then juice the remaining part of the cucumber. Stir ingredients, pour into a glass, and drink as soon as possible.

SERVES 1

MINT REFRESHER

2 stalks fennel with leaves
1/2 cucumber, peeled
1/2 green apple such
    as Granny Smith or
    pippin

1 small handful mint
1-inch chunk gingerroot,
    scrubbed, or peeled
    if old

Cut produce to fit your juicer's feed tube. Juice ingredients and stir. Pour into a glass and drink as soon as possible.

SERVES 1 TO 2

MAGNESIUM-RICH BLEND

3 to 4 carrots, scrubbed
    well, tops removed,
    ends trimmed
2 celery stalks, with leaves
    as desired

1/2 small beet, scrubbed
    well, with 1 or 2 leaves
2 to 3 broccoli florets
1/2 lemon, peeled

Cut produce to fit your juicer's feed tube. Juice ingredients and stir. Pour into a glass and drink as soon as possible.

SERVES 1

BEAUTIFUL-SKIN COCKTAIL

1 cucumber, peeled   *1/2 lemon, peeled*
1 parsnip, peeled   *1/4 green bell pepper*
2 to 3 carrots, scrubbed
*   well, tops removed,*
*   ends trimmed*

Cut produce to fit your juicer's feed tube. Juice ingredients and stir. Pour into a glass and drink as soon as possible.
SERVES 1 TO 2

Note: Cucumber and bell pepper are good sources of the trace mineral silicon, which is recommended to strengthen skin, hair, and fingernails along with bones. In studies, silicon has been shown to reduce signs of aging such as improving thickness of skin and reducing wrinkles.

CALCIUM-RICH COCKTAIL

1 cucumber, peeled   *1/2 lemon, peeled*
1 to 2 medium to large   *1-inch chunk gingerroot,*
*   kale leaves*   *   scrubbed, or peeled*
1 handful parsley   *   if old*
1 celery stalk

Cut produce to fit your juicer's feed tube. Juice ingredients and stir. Pour into a glass and drink as soon as possible.
SERVES 1 TO 2

Note: Kale and parsley are high in calcium.

PEPPY PARSLEY

1 bunch parsley
2 celery stalks
1 to 2 carrots, scrubbed
    well, tops removed,
    ends trimmed

1/2 cucumber, peeled
1/2 lemon, peeled

Cut produce to fit your juicer's feed tube. Juice ingredients and stir. Pour into a glass and drink as soon as possible.
SERVES 1

THE REVITALIZER

2 tomatoes
1/2 cucumber, peeled
6 to 8 string beans

1/2 lemon or lime, peeled
Dash of hot sauce

Cut produce to fit your juicer's feed tube. Juice ingredients and stir. Pour into a glass and drink as soon as possible.
SERVES 1

WEIGHT-LOSS HELPER

1 small Jerusalem
    artichoke (sun choke),
    scrubbed well
3 to 4 carrots, scrubbed
    well, tops removed,
    ends trimmed

1/2 small beet, scrubbed
    well, with 1 or 2 leaves

Cut produce to fit your juicer's feed tube. Juice ingredients and stir. Pour into a glass and drink as soon as possible.
SERVES 1

Note: Jerusalem artichoke has a substance known as inulin that prolongs carbohydrate metabolism, which helps appetite control. It's also been used to improve liver function, which helps weight loss. The key is to sip it slowly when you get a craving for high-fat or high-carb foods.

GOOD SLEEP NIGHTCAP

2 romaine lettuce leaves
1 small handful parsley
1/2 cucumber, peeled
3 carrots, scrubbed well,
tops removed, ends
    trimmed
1 stalk celery

Bunch up the parsley and roll in a romaine leaf. Juice the cucumber and turn off the machine. Add the romaine and parsley, turn the machine back on, and tap it through with a carrot. Juice remaining produce, stir the juice, and drink as soon as possible.

SERVES 1

MOOD MENDER

3 fennel stalks, including
    leaves and flowers
3 carrots, scrubbed well,
    tops removed, ends
    trimmed
2 stalks celery
1/2 pear
1/2-inch chunk
    gingerroot, scrubbed,
    or peeled if old

Cut produce to fit your juicer's feed tube. Juice ingredients and stir. Pour into a glass and drink as soon as possible.

SERVES 1 TO 2

Note: Fennel juice has been used as a traditional tonic to help the body release endorphins, the "feel good" peptides, from the brain into the bloodstream. Endorphins help to diminish anxiety and fear and generate a mood of euphoria.

HEALTHY SINUS SOLUTION

2 vine-ripened tomatoes   6 radishes, scrubbed
1/2 cucumber, peeled   1/2 lime, peeled

Cut produce to fit your juicer's feed tube. Juice ingredients and stir. Pour into a glass and drink as soon as possible.
SERVES 1

Note: Radish juice is a traditional remedy for opening up the sinuses and supporting the mucus membranes.

THE IMMUNE SUPPORTER

1 handful watercress   pippin or 1/2 lemon,
1 turnip, scrubbed, tops   peeled
    removed, ends trimmed   3 carrots, scrubbed well,
1 to 2 garlic cloves   tops removed, ends
1/2 green apple such   trimmed
    as Granny Smith or

Bunch up watercress. Cut produce to fit your juicer's feed tube. Tuck the watercress in the feed tube and push through with the turnip. Juice remaining ingredients, finishing with a carrot. Stir the juice, pour into a glass, and drink as soon as possible.
SERVES 1

Note: Studies show that garlic has a compound that has a natural antibiotic-like effect, and is very helpful for the immune system. It is antibacterial, antifungal, antiparasitic, and antiviral, but it must be consumed raw to have this effect.

PANCREAS-HELPER COCKTAIL

2 romaine leaves
1/2 cucumber, peeled
1 large vine-ripened
   tomato

8 to 10 string beans
2 Brussels sprouts
1/2 lemon, peeled

Bunch up romaine leaves. Cut produce to fit your juicer's feed tube. Tuck the romaine in the feed tube and push through with the cucumber. Juice remaining ingredients, finishing with some tomato. Pour into a glass and drink as soon as possible.

SERVES 1

Note: Brussels sprouts and string bean juice have been used as traditional remedies to help strengthen and support the pancreas. Drink before a meal. (If this drink is too strong, dilute with a little water.) For best pancreas support, also avoid refined carbohydrates such as white flour products, sugars of all type, soda pop, and all sweets.

HEALTHY-LUNG SOLUTION

1 handful watercress
1 small turnip, scrubbed
   well, tops removed,
   ends trimmed
2-inch-thick chunk of
   jicama, scrubbed well
   or peeled

2 to 3 carrots, scrubbed
   well, tops removed,
   ends trimmed
1 garlic clove
1/2 lemon, peeled

Bunch up watercress. Cut produce to fit your juicer's feed tube. Tuck the watercress in feed tube and push through with the turnip. Juice remaining ingredients, finishing with a carrot. Stir the juice, pour into a glass, and drink as soon as possible.

SERVES 1

Note: Turnip juice has been used as a traditional remedy to strengthen lung tissue.

Smoothies, Blender Drinks, and Cold Soups

CHERIE'S GREEN DELIGHT

1/2 English cucumber, peeled and cut in chunks
1 avocado, peeled and seeded and cut in quarters
1 cup raw spinach

1/2 to 3/4 cup coconut milk*
Juice of 1 lime
1 tablespoon green powder of choice (optional)
2 to 3 tablespoons ground almonds (optional)

Combine all ingredients in a blender and blend well. Sprinkle ground almonds on top, as desired.
SERVES 2

ENERGY SOUP

2 to 3 carrots, scrubbed, tops removed, ends trimmed
2 to 3 stalks celery
1/2 cucumber, peeled
1/2 lemon, peeled and seeded
Handful of parsley

1- to 2-inch chunk gingerroot, peeled
1 avocado
Garnish options: grated zucchini, fresh corn, or crunchy sprouts such as pea, lentil, and bean

---

*The best coconut milk can be found in plastic pouches in the frozen section of Asian stores. A great brand is Anahaw, distributed by Ferntrade.

Juice the carrots, celery, cucumber, lemon, parsley, and gingerroot. Pour the juice into a blender and add the avocado. Blend until smooth. Pour into bowls and serve immediately. You may garnish with any of the optional additions for a crunchy topper.

SERVES 2

YUMMY BROCCOLI SOUP

1 cup vegetable stock
1 to 2 cups broccoli,
     chopped
1/2 onion, chopped
1 red or yellow bell
     pepper, chopped
1 to 2 stalks celery,
     chopped

1 avocado, peeled and
     seeded
Bragg Liquid Aminos or
     sea salt to taste
Cumin or grated ginger
     to taste
Lemon (optional)

Gently warm the vegetable stock, keeping the temperature at or below 118°F.* Add the broccoli and onion and warm for 5 minutes. Turn off heat. Then add the bell pepper and celery for an additional 5 minutes.

Puree the broccoli, onion, bell pepper, and celery with the vegetable broth in a blender until smooth. Add the avocado and blend until smooth.

Add Bragg Liquid Aminos or sea salt to taste. If using cumin, add and blend.

If using grated ginger, add to the top of the soup and stir in.

A squeeze of lemon is nice. Add as desired.

SERVES 2

---

*At 118°F or below, the vitamins and enzymes are not destroyed; it's considered raw food.

SPICY YAM BISQUE

1 cup yam juice
1 cup sesame, almond, or
   rice milk
1/4 cup red onion, chopped
1 avocado, peeled and
   seeded

1 teaspoon nutmeg
1/4 teaspoon cinnamon
1/4 teaspoon ground allspice
1/4 teaspoon ground mace
1/4 teaspoon cardamom

Juice 1 cup of yam juice. Let it sit until the starch settles to the bottom of the measuring cup. This should take about an hour. Pour off the clear juice, but not the starchy portion as this will make the soup gritty.

Pour the yam juice and milk of choice in a blender. Add the onion and avocado and blend until smooth. Add the spices and blend.

SERVES 2

THE HEALTHY NUT

1 cup unsweetened
   pineapple juice (juice
   about 1/4 small
   pineapple, if making
   fresh juice)
10 almonds, whole or
   blanched
1 tablespoon sunflower
   seeds
1 tablespoon sesame
   seeds

1 tablespoon flaxseed
1 tablespoon chia seeds
   (optional)
1 cup chopped parsley
1/2 cup almond, rice, or
   sesame milk
1/2 teaspoon pure vanilla
   extract
1 tablespoon protein
   powder
6 ice cubes

Place the pineapple juice, nuts, and seeds in a bowl, cover, and soak overnight. Place this nut and seed mixture with the juice in the blender and add the parsley, milk, vanilla, protein powder, and ice cubes. Blend on high speed until smooth. This smoothie will be a bit chewy because of the nuts and seeds. It makes a great breakfast.

To kill molds, when soaking nuts and seeds, add 1/2 teaspoon ascorbic acid to the pineapple juice.

SERVES 2

SPINACH-AVOCADO SOUP

1 avocado

1 cucumber, peeled, cut in chunks

1 small jalapeño, seeded

Juice of 1/2 to 1 lemon

1/2 cup water

1 to 2 cloves garlic

1 tablespoon cilantro

1 tablespoon fresh parsley

1/4 purple onion, finely chopped (for garnish)

Place all ingredients in a blender or food processor and puree until smooth. Pour into a bowl and add chopped onion, or any other chopped vegetables or herbs, as a garnish.

SERVES 2

CREAMY TOMATO SOUP

1/2 large avocado or 1 small avocado

1 to 2 vine-ripened tomatoes

2 tablespoons chopped sweet red bell pepper

1/4 carrot, chopped in small pieces

3/4 cup sesame or almond milk

Combine all ingredients in a blender and blend well. Pour into bowls.

SERVES 2

SUMMER CORN CHOWDER

2 cups fresh or frozen corn
  kernels (about 2 large
  ears)
1 cup almond milk
1 avocado, cut in chunks
1/4 red bell pepper, cut in
  chunks
2 teaspoons chopped
  onion

1/2 teaspoon ground
  cumin
1/2 teaspoon sea salt
Garnish: 1 tablespoon
  each, chopped parsley
  and minced red bell
  pepper (optional)

In a blender, combine the corn, almond milk, avocado, bell
pepper, onion, cumin, and salt. Blend well. Pour into bowls
and garnish with parsley and red pepper.

SERVES 2

MINTY CUCUMBER SOUP

1 cucumber, peeled and
  cut into chunks
1 avocado, cut in chunks

1/4 cup chopped fresh
  mint

Combine all ingredients in a blender and blend well. Pour
into a bowl.

SERVES 1

GARDEN TOMATO SOUP

3 small tomatoes or 2
   medium
2 green onions (about
   2 inches of tips and
   green) chopped

1/2 green pepper, chopped
1 cup vegetable broth
1 avocado
1 teaspoon sea salt

Combine all ingredients in a blender and blend well. Pour into bowls.

SERVES 2

FRENCH TOMATO-BASIL SOUP

6 medium tomatoes
1/2 lemon, peeled, seeded,
   and cut into chunks
1 avocado
2 tablespoons chopped
   fresh basil

1 tablespoon chopped
   onion
1 small garlic clove
Basil leaves for garnish

In a blender, blend the tomatoes until chunky. Add the lemon, avocado, basil, onion, and garlic. Blend well. Pour into bowls and garnish with fresh basil leaves.

SERVES 2

HEARTY KALE SOUP

3 large kale leaves
3 stalks celery
1/2 lemon, peeled

1 avocado
1 cup spinach leaves

Juice the kale, celery, and lemon. Pour into a blender, add the avocado and spinach and blend well. Pour into bowls and serve.

SERVES 2

VEGETABLE HARVEST SOUP

2 cups water or vegetable
  broth
1 cup green beans,
  chopped
1 cup asparagus, chopped
2 carrots, chopped
2 stalks celery, chopped
1/2 onion, chopped

2 cups water or vegetable
  broth
Pinch of mace
1 teaspoon sea salt
1 tablespoon chopped
  parsley for garnish

Pour water or vegetable broth into a soup pot. Add the vegetables and gently warm for about 10 minutes, or until vegetables are just slightly tender. Pour ingredients with the water or vegetable broth into a blender, add the mace and sea salt, and blend well. Pour into bowls and garnish with parsley.

SERVES 2

SPINACH POWER SOUP

1 avocado
1/2 cup water
1 cucumber, peeled and
  cut in chunks
1 green onion, chopped
1/4 red bell pepper,
  chopped

1 clove garlic, chopped
1/2 teaspoon sea salt
1 cup spinach
Raw pumpkin seeds for
  garnish

Combine the avocado and water in a blender and blend well. Add the cucumber, green onion, bell pepper, garlic, and salt. Blend well. Add the spinach and blend well. Pour into bowls. Garnish with pumpkin seeds.

SERVES 2

ZIPPY ASPARAGUS SOUP

10 stalks asparagus,
    chopped
4 tomatoes, cut in chunks
1/4 cup water
1/4 cup fresh parsley,
    chopped
1/4 cup chopped onion
1/2 red bell pepper,
    chopped

3 to 4 sundried tomatoes
2 cloves garlic
1/2 teaspoon sea salt or
    Bragg Liquid Aminos
1 avocado
1/2 lemon (cut in quarters)

Combine asparagus, tomatoes, water, parsley, onion, bell pepper, sundried tomatoes, garlic, and salt in a blender and blend well. Add the avocado and blend well. Pour into bowls and add a squeeze of lemon to each bowl.

SERVES 2

REFRESHING TOMATILLO CUCUMBER SOUP

1 cucumber, peeled and
    cut in chunks
2 tomatillos
1 lime (peeled and
    seeded), cut in chunks

2 cups fresh spinach
1/2 cup almond milk
1 avocado
4 to 6 ice cubes

Combine the cucumber, tomatillos, lime, spinach, and almond milk in a blender and blend well. Add the avocado and ice cubes and blend well. Pour into bowls.

SERVES 2

CREAMY CAULIFLOWER SOUP

1/2 onion, chopped
3 stalks celery, chopped
1 head cauliflower,
    chopped
1 tablespoon virgin
    coconut oil

1 cup almond milk
1/2 teaspoon sea salt
Pepper to taste (optional)

Lightly steam onion, celery, and cauliflower for about 5 minutes or until just tender. Combine in a blender with the coconut oil, almond milk, salt, and pepper as desired. Blend well. Pour into bowls.

SERVES 2

ZIPPY TOMATO SOUP

2 radishes, scrubbed
2 stalks celery
1/2 lemon, peeled
2 tomatoes, chopped
1 garlic clove, peeled
1 to 2 pickled umebushi
    plums, seeds removed

1/2 teaspoon freshly
    grated lemon peel,
    preferably organic
Dash of cayenne pepper
4 to 6 ice cubes

Juice the radishes, celery, and lemon. Pour the juices into a blender and add the tomatoes, garlic, umebushi plums, lemon peel, cayenne, and ice. Blend on high speed until smooth, pour into bowls, and serve immediately.

SERVES 1 TO 2

SIMPLY REFRESHING SHAKE

*1/2 cucumber, peeled and
    cut in chunks
1 stalk celery, juiced or
    chopped into small
    pieces
Juice of 1/2 lemon*

*1/2 teaspoon freshly
    grated lemon peel,
    preferably organic
1/2 teaspoon ascorbic acid
    (vitamin C powder)
Nutritional yeast (optional)*

Place the cucumber chunks in a freezer bag and freeze them until solid. Combine the frozen cucumber chunks in a blender with the celery, lemon juice, lemon peel, and ascorbic acid. Blend on high speed until smooth, sprinkle with nutritional yeast as desired, and serve immediately.

SERVES 1

COCONUT SHAKE

*1 cup coconut milk
1 tablespoon virgin
    coconut oil
1 tablespoon ground
    flaxseeds
1 teaspoon pure vanilla
    extract*

*1/4 teaspoon almond
    extract
1/4 teaspoon stevia
    powder
8 to 10 ice cubes*

Place all ingredients but ice in a blender and process at high speed until well combined. Add ice after the coconut oil is blended so that it won't clump. You may use more or less ice, depending on how cold you like a smoothie.

SERVES 1 TO 2

TOMATO WITH A TWIST

2 tomatoes, cut in chunks
1 cup tomato juice (2 to
    3 medium tomatoes,
    juiced)
1/2 lemon, juiced

1 teaspoon freshly grated
    lemon rind, preferably
    organic
6 fresh basil leaves, rinsed

Place the tomato chunks in a freezer bag and freeze them until solid. Pour the tomato juice into a blender and add the frozen tomato chunks, lemon juice, lemon peel, and basil. Blend on high speed until smooth and serve immediately.

SERVES 1

ICY SPICY TOMATO

2 tomatoes, cut in chunks
1 cup fresh carrot juice
    (about 5 to 7 carrots)
1/2 lemon, juiced, peeled
    if using a juice
    machine
2 tablespoons cilantro,
    rinsed and chopped

1/4 teaspoon sea salt
1/4 teaspoon ground
    cumin
1/4 small jalapeño,
    chopped, or to taste
3 radishes, washed and
    chopped

Place the tomato chunks in a freezer bag and freeze them until solid. Pour the carrot and lemon juices into a blender and add the frozen tomato chunks, cilantro, salt, cumin, jalapeño, and radishes. Blend on high speed until smooth and serve immediately.

SERVES 1

SALSA SHAKE

2 cups tomato, cut in
    chunks
1 cup fresh cucumber
    juice (1/2 cucumber,
    peeled if not organic,
    and juiced, or peeled,
    cut in chunks, and
    frozen)

1 lemon, juiced
1/2 teaspoon freshly
    grated lemon peel,
    preferably organic
2 daikon radishes, washed
    (optional)
Dash cayenne pepper

Place tomato chunks (and cucumber if freezing) in a freezer bag and freeze them until solid. Pour the cucumber juice or place frozen cucumber chunks and the lemon juice into a blender and add the frozen tomato chunks, lemon peel, daikon radishes, if using, and cayenne. Blend on high speed until smooth and serve immediately.

SERVES 1 TO 2

CREAMY TOMATO COOLER

2 cups tomatoes, washed
    and chopped
1 avocado, chopped
1/2 cup almond or sesame
    milk
1/2 teaspoon freshly
    grated lemon peel,
    preferably organic

1/2 teaspoon balsamic
    vinegar
1/2 lemon, juiced
Dash of cayenne pepper
    (optional)

Place the tomato chunks in a freezer bag and freeze until solid. Combine the tomato chunks, avocado, milk, lemon peel, balsamic vinegar, lemon juice, and cayenne as desired in a blender. Blend on high speed until smooth and serve immediately.

SERVES 1 TO 2

CARROT-TOMATO COOLER

3 medium tomatoes, cut
    into chunks
1 1/2 cups fresh carrot juice
    (about 6 large carrots)
1 tablespoon balsamic
    vinegar or fresh lemon
    juice

2 teaspoons tamari or
    Bragg Liquid Aminos
1 garlic clove, peeled
Garnish: finely chopped
    cilantro or parsley

Place the tomato chunks in a freezer bag and freeze them until solid. Pour the carrot juice, balsamic vinegar or lemon juice, and tamari or Bragg Liquid Aminos in a blender and add the tomato chunks and garlic; blend on high speed until smooth. Garnish as desired and serve immediately.
SERVES 2

CUCUMBER-AVOCADO SOUP

1 1/4 cups fresh cucumber
    juice (about l large or
    2 medium cucumbers,
    peeled if not organic)
2 stalks celery, juiced
1 avocado
1 garlic clove, peeled

1/2 cup almond milk
1/2 cup parsley, coarsely
    chopped
2 teaspoons onion,
    chopped
1 teaspoon dried dill weed

Pour the cucumber and celery juices into a blender and add the avocado, garlic, milk, parsley, onion, and dill. Blend on high speed until smooth and serve immediately. This soup is not good if it sits.
SERVES 2

CREAMY RED PEPPER SOUP

3 large red bell peppers
6 garlic cloves
1 cup almond milk
1 tablespoon balsamic
vinegar

2 teaspoons tamari or
Bragg Liquid Aminos
6 fresh basil leaves, rinsed
Garnish: chopped fresh
basil (optional)

Lightly steam the peppers and garlic for about 5 minutes or just until tender. Cut the peppers into chunks. Pour the milk into a blender and add the peppers, garlic, balsamic vinegar, tamari or Bragg Liquid Aminos, and basil. Blend on high speed until smooth. Pour into bowls and garnish with fresh basil, as desired. Serve immediately.

SERVES 1 TO 2

CUCUMBER-MINT SOUP

1 cup almond milk
2 cups cucumber, peeled
and diced
1/4 cup scallions, chopped

1/2 teaspoon sea salt
6 mint leaves
1 garlic clove, peeled and
minced

Combine the milk with the cucumber, scallions, salt, mint, and garlic in a blender and process on high speed until smooth. Pour into bowls and serve immediately.

SERVES 2

Resources Guide

WEB SITES FOR CHERIE AND JOHN CALBOM

www.juicelife.com

www.sleepawaythepounds.com: information about the Sleep Away the Pounds program and products

www.gococonuts.com: information about *The Coconut Diet* and coconut oil

www.cheriecalbom.com: information about the authors and their books and other Web sites

OTHER BOOKS BY CHERIE AND JOHN CALBOM

Note: These books can be ordered at any of the Web sites noted above or through 866-843-8935

Sleep Away the Pounds (Warner Wellness) by Cherie Calbom and John Calbom

The Wrinkle Cleanse (Avery) by Cherie Calbom

The Coconut Diet (Warner Books) by Cherie Calbom and John Calbom

The Complete Cancer Cleanse (Warner Books) by Cherie Calbom, John Calbom, and Michael Mahaffey

The Ultimate Smoothie Book (Warner Books) by Cherie Calbom

The Juice Lady's Guide to Juicing for Health rev. ed. (Avery) by Cherie Calbom

JUICERS

Find out the best juicers recommended by Cherie.
Call 866-8GETWEL (1-866-843-8935) or visit the Web site www.juicelife.com

LYMPHASIZER

Call 866-8GETWEL (866-843-8935) or visit the Web site www.juicelife.com

FOOD PRODUCTS

Coconut oil: Call 866-8GETWEL (866-843-8935) or visit the Web site www.juicelife.com to order virgin coconut oil

CLEANSE PRODUCTS

OVERALL CLEANSE

Silver Creek Labs Creation's Cleanse; 800-493-1146

COLON CLEANSE PRODUCTS

Advanced Naturals: Fiber Max, Colon Cleanse I and II (available at health food stores)

Arise & Shine Products: Psyllium, Bentonite, Herbal Nutrition, and Chomper; 888-557-4463

Blessed Herbs; 800-489-4372; www.blessedherbs.com

Dr. Schultz Colon Cleanse Products Formula I & II; 877-832-2463

Silver Creek Labs Colon Cleanser Complete; 800-493-1146

LIVER CLEANSE PRODUCTS

Chinese herbal tinctures (four-part kit) to use with Cherie's Liver Detox Program; 866-843-8935

Dr. Schultz's 5-Day Liver Detox Kit; 877-832-2463

S.A.T. (milk thistle, artichoke, turmeric) Thorne; 866-843-8935

CANDIDA ALBICANS CLEANSE PRODUCTS

Fungal Defense — Garden of Life; www.gardenoflifeusa.com; 800-622-8986

Yeast Max — Advanced Naturals (health food stores)

Silver Creek Labs Candida Cleanse; 800-493-1146

Candidaise — health food stores

HCL with pepsin; 866-843-8935

You can order a stool test at www.gdx.net or www.great plainslaboratory.com.

PARASITE CLEANSE PRODUCTS

Worm Squirm I and II — Arise & Shine; 888-557-4463

Silver Creek Labs ParaCease & ParaAssist; 800-493-1146

Ness Formula (systemic enzymes); 866-843-8935

You can order a parasite test at www.gdx.net or www.great plainslaboratory.com.

KIDNEY CLEANSE HERBS

Arise & Shine Kidney Life; 888-557-4463

Dr. Schultz's Kidney Cleanse Detox Kit; 877-832-2463

HEAVY METAL CLEANSE

Arise & Shine; 888-557-4463

HEALTH CENTERS UTILIZING JUICE AND RAW FOODS CLEANSE PROGRAMS

The following centers offer a raw foods and/or juice detoxification program. Most of them offer nutritional classes and some offer other health classes that address the emotional, mental, and spiritual aspects of health and renewal. Most of the centers also offer massage and colonics. It is best to contact the various centers to find out which one best fits your needs:

Cedar Springs Renewal Center
Michael Mahaffey and Nan Monk, Directors
31459 Barben Road
Sedro Woolley, WA 98284
(360) 826-3599
fax: (360) 422-1524
Web site: www.cedarsprings.org

HealthQuarters Ministries
David Frahm, ND, Director
3620 W. Colorado Avenue
Colorado Springs, CO 80904
(719) 593-8694
fax: (719) 531-7884
e-mail: healthqu@healthquarters.org
Web site: www.healthquarters.org

Hippocrates Institute
Brian and Anna Maria Clement, Directors
1443 Palmdale Court
West Palm Beach, FL 33411
(800) 842-2125
fax: (561) 471-9464
e-mail: hippocrates@worldnet.att.net
Web site: www.hippocratesinstitute.org

Monastery Wellness Institute
Fr. John and Cherie Calbom, Directors
Vashon Island, WA 98070
(866) 843-8935

Optimum Health Institute of Austin
Route 1 Box 339 J
Cedar Creek, TX 78612
(512) 303-4817
fax: (512) 303-1239
e-mail: austin@optimumhealth.org
Web site: www.optimumhealth.org

Optimum Health Institute of San Diego
6970 Central Avenue
Lemon Grove, CA 91945
(800) 993-4325
fax: (619) 589-4098
e-mail: optimum@optimumhealth.org
Web site: www.optimumhealth.org

Sanoviv Medical Institute
Dr. Myron Wentz, Director
Playa de Rosarito, Km 39
Baja California, Mexico
(800) 726-6848
fax: (801) 954-7477
Web site: www.sanoviv.com

We Care
Susana and Susan Lombardi, Directors
18000 Long Canyon Road
Desert Hot Springs, CA 92241
(800) 888-2523
fax: (760) 251-5399
e-mail: info@wecarespa.com
Web site: www.wecarespa.com

References

CHAPTER ONE

Anderson, Richard. *The Liver: Cleansing and Rejuvenating the Vital Organ.* Medford, OR: Christobe Publishing, 1999.

Baker, Arthur M. "Raw Fresh Produce vs. Cooked Food." http://www.rawfoodlife.com.

BBC News online, "Organic Food 'Proven' Healthier," January 3, 2000. http://www. news.bbc.co.uk/1/hi/sci/tech/588589.stm.

Calbom, Cherie, and John Calbom. *The Coconut Diet.* New York: Warner, 2005.

Calbom, Cherie, John Calbom, and Michael Mahaffey. *The Complete Cancer Cleanse.* Nashville, TN: Thomas Nelson, 2003.

Cornforth, Tracee. "Environmental Toxins and Reproductive Health." *Your Guide to Women's Health.* http://womens health.about.com/cs/azhealthtopics/a/envtoxrephealth .htm

Cross, C.E., et al. "Oxygen radicals and human diseases." *Annals of Internal Medicine* 107 (1987): 526.

Harman, D. "Free radical theory of aging: role of free radicals in the origination and evolution of life, aging, and disease processes." In *Free Radicals, Aging and Degenerative Diseases,* edited by J. E. Johnson, 3–50. New York: Alan R. Liss, 1986.

Koebnick, Corinna, et al. "Long-Term Consumption of a Raw Food Diet Is Associated with Favorable Serum LDL Cholesterol and Triglycerides but also with Elevated Plasma Homocysteine and Low Serum HDL Cholesterol in Humans." *Journal of Nutrition* 122, no. 4 (April 1992): 924–30.

Mayeda, Andrew. "Test finds MPs' bodies full of toxins." *Vancouver Sun* online, January 4, 2007. http://www.canada .com/vancouversun/news/story.html?id=7ccc417c-e082 -40ac-a203-303e288c2cb9&k=19093

Mercola, Joseph, M.D. "Scientists Warn: Dangerous Chemicals Found in Plastic." http://articles.mercola.com/sites/ articles/archive/2007/08/07/scientists-warn-of-the-dangers -of-a-chemical-found-in-plastic.aspx.

———. "The Truth About Tap Water." http://articles.mercola .com/sites/articles/archive/2007/08/06/the-truth-about -tap-water.aspx.

Schneider, Andrew. "That Buttery Aroma Might Be Toxic, Too." *Seattle Post Intelligencer,* August 30, 2007.

Sinatra, Stephen, M.D. "Toxin Exposure in Infancy Affects Health for a Lifetime." *Heart, Health, and Nutrition* newsletter, August 2007: 2–4.

U.S. Centers for Disease Control and Prevention (CDC). "National Report on Human Exposure to Environmental Chemicals." July 21, 2005. http://www.cdc.gov/exposure report/default.htm.

U.S. Environmental Protection Agency. "Endocrine Disruptor Screening Program." 1996. http://www.epa.gov/scipoly/ oscpendo/pubs/edspoverview/background.htm.

U.S. Food and Drug Administration, Center for Biologics Evaluation and Research. "Thimerosal in Vaccines." http:// www.fda.gov/cber/vaccine/thimerosal.htm.

Vandenberg, Laura N., Russ Hauser, Michele Marcus, Nicolas Olea, and Wade V. Welshons. "Human Exposure to Bisphenol A (BPA)." *Human Toxicology* 25 (July 2007).

CHAPTER TWO

Appel, L. J., T. J. Moore, E. Obarzanek, et al. "A clinical trial of the effects of dietary patterns on blood pressure." DASH Collaborative Research Group. *New England Journal of Medicine* 336 (1997): 1117–24.

"Aspartame and Dieting," *Nutrition Week* 27, no. 23 (June 13, 1997); *International Journal of Obesity* 21, no. 1 (January 1997): 37–42.

Brown, L., E. B. Rimm, J. M. Seddon, et al. "A prospective study of carotenoid intake and risk of cataract extraction in U.S. men." *American Journal of Clinical Nutrition* 70 (1999): 517–24.

Calbom, Cherie, M.S. *The Juice Lady's Guide to Juicing for Health.* New York: Avery, 1999.

———. *The Juice Lady's Juicing for High Level Wellness and Vibrant Good Looks.* New York: Three Rivers Press, 1999.

"Cancer and Tomatoes," *Nutrition Week* 7 (December 15, 1995). Taken from December 6, 1995, issue of *Journal of the National Cancer Institute.*

Center for Nutrition Policy and Promotion. "2005 Dietary Guidelines for Americans." U.S. Department of Agriculture.

Checkbiotech.org. "Hungary hopeful it can keep its GMO ban." www.checkbiotech.org.

Cheney, G., et al. "Anti-Peptic Ulcer Dietary Factor (Vitamin 'U') in the Treatment of Peptic Ulcers." *Journal of the American Dietetic Association* 25 (1950): 668–72.

Cho, E., J. M. Seddon, B. Rosner, W. C. Willett, and S. E. Hankinson. "Prospective study of intake of fruits, vegetables, vitamins, and carotenoids and risk of age-related maculopathy." *Archives of Ophthalmology* 122 (2004): 883–92.

Djousse, L., D. K. Arnett, H. Coon, M. A. Province, L. L. Moore, and R. C. Ellison. "Fruit and vegetable consumption and LDL cholesterol: The National Heart, Lung, and Blood

Institute Family Heart Study." *American Journal of Clinical Nutrition* 79 (2004): 213–7.

Environmental Working Group. "Food News: Shopper's Guide," 5th edition. Data are from the USFDA between 2000 and 2005. http://www.foodnews.org/index.php.

FoodNavigator-USA.com. "Pure juices can reduce disease risk." http://www.foodnavigator-usa.com/news/ng.asp?n=73732-alltracel-provexis-juice-drinks. H9/07

Gupta, Chris. "Nutrition and Cooking/Freezing." September 24, 2005. http://www.newmediaexplorer.org/chris/2003/10/18/nutrition_and_cookingfreezing.htm.

Harvard School of Public Health. "Food Pyramids." http://www.hsph.harvard.edu/nutritionsource/pyramids.html.

Hung, H. C., K. J. Joshipura, R. Jiang, et al. "Fruit and vegetable intake and risk of major chronic disease." *Journal of National Cancer Institute* 96 (2004): 1577–84.

Kjeldsen-Kragh, J., et al. "Controlled Trial of Fasting and One Year Vegetarian Diet in Rheumatoid Arthritis." *The Lancet* 338 (October 12, 1991): 899–902.

Krinsky, N. I., J. T. Landrum, R. A. Bone. "Biologic mechanisms of the protective role of lutein and zeaxanthin in the eye." *Annual Review of Nutrition* 23 (2003): 171–201.

Mayo Clinic staff. "Macular Degeneration." August 2006. http://www.mayoclinic.com/health/macular-degeneration/DS00284.

Mercola, Joseph, M.D. "Even Mice Don't Like Genetically Modified Food." January 2002. http://www.mercola.com/2002/jan/23/gm_food.htm.

———. "How Do You Know If Your Food Is Genetically Modified?" http://www.mercola.com/2004/jan/24/gm_foods.htm.

———. "GM Corn Causes Organ Damage in Rats: Will It Cause It in You?" http://v.mercola.com/blogs/public_blog/GM-Corn-Causes-Organ-Damage-in-Rats—Will-It-Cause-It-In-You—7892.aspx.

————. "Liquid Candy Becoming the Preferred Breakfast Drink." February 1, 2007. http://www.mercola.com/2007/feb/1/liquid-candy-becoming-the-preferred-breakfast-drink.htm.

Moeller, S. M., A. Taylor, K. L. Tucker, et al. "Overall adherence to the dietary guidelines for Americans is associated with reduced prevalence of early age-related nuclear lens opacities in women." *Journal of Nutrition* 134 (2004): 1812–9.

Morse, Robert, N.D. *The Detox Miracle Sourcebook.* Prescott, AZ: Holm Press, 2004.

ScientificAmerican.com. "GMO corn causes liver, kidney problems in rats: study." March 13, 2007. http://www.sciam.com/article.cfm?alias=gmo-corn-causes-liver-kid&chanId=sa013.

Séralini, Gilles-Eric, et al. "New Analysis of a Rat Feeding Study with a Genetically Modified Maize Reveals Signs of Hepatorenal Toxicity." *Archives of Environmental Contamination and Toxicology,* March 14, 2007. http://www.springerlink.com/content/02648wu132m07804/?p=a4782763081842a38c67449a8b48e6d3&pi=6

Tortora, Gerard J., Sandra R. Grabowski. *Introduction to the Human Body: The Essentials of Anatomy and Physiology,* sixth edition. Hoboken, NJ: John Wiley & Sons, 2004.

Tsang, Gloria, R.D. "Fiber 101: Soluble Fiber vs. Insoluble Fiber Benefits of Fiber." Healthcastle.com, November 2005. http://www.healthcastle.com/fiber-solubleinsoluble.shtml.

U.S. Centers for Disease Control and Prevention (CDC). "Fruits and Vegetables." http://www.cdc.gov/nccdphp/dnpa/nutrition/nutrition_for_everyone/quick_tips/fruit_vegetable.htm.

————. "Do you eat enough fruits and vegetables?" http://www.fruitsandveggiesmatter.gov/spotlight.html

Vainio, H., and F. Bianchini. *IARC Handbooks of Cancer Prevention: Fruit and Vegetables,* vol. 8. Lyon, France: IARC, 2003.

Wikipedia. "Dietary Fiber." http://en.wikipedia.org/wiki/ Dietary_fiber.

Young, Emma. "GM pea causes allergic damage in mice." NewScientist.com, November 21, 2005. http://www.new scientist.com/article.ns?id=dn8347.

CHAPTER THREE

"Alkalinity." www.snyderhealth.com/alkalinity.htm.

Calbom, Cherie, M.S. *The Juice Lady's Juicing for High Level Wellness and Vibrant Good Looks.* New York: Three Rivers Press, 1999.

————. *The Juice Lady's Guide to Juicing for Health.* New York: Avery, 1999.

Colbert, Don, M.D. *Toxic Relief: Restore Health and Energy Through Fasting and Detoxification.* Lake Mary, FL: Siloam, 2001 and 2003.

Floyd, Ronnie W. *The Power of Prayer and Fasting: 19 Secret of Spiritual Strength.* Nashville, TN: Broadman & Holman, 1997.

Fourest-Fontecave, S., U. Adamson, P. E. Lins, B. Ekblom, C. Sandahl, and L. Strand. "Mental alertness in response to hypoglycaemia in normal man: the effect of 12 hours and 72 hours of fasting." NCBI PubMed/*Diabète et métabolisme* 13, no. 4 (July–August 1987): 405–10. http://www .ncbi.nlm.nih.gov/entrez/query.fcgi?cmd=Retrieve&db =PubMed&list_uids=3315761&dopt=Abstract.

Lagerquist, Ron. *Fasting to Freedom: A Revolution of Body and Spirit,* revised ed. Sunderland, ON: Renewed Health, 2003.

————. http://www.freedomyou.com.

Mercola, Joseph, M.D. http://www.mercola.com.

Morse, Robert, N.D. *The Detox Miracle Sourcebook.* Prescott, AZ: Holm Press, 2004.

Sewald, Peter. *Wisdom of the Monastery.* Old Saybrook, CT: Konecky & Konecky, 2003.

Shelton, H. M. *Fasting Can Save Your Life*, fourth printing. Bridgeport, CT: American Natural Hygiene Society Inc., 1964, 1978, and 1991.

CHAPTER FOUR

Anderson, Richard. *The Liver: Cleansing and Rejuvenating the Vital Organ*. Medford, OR: Christobe Publishing, 1999.

Calbom, Cherie, and John Calbom. *The Coconut Diet*. New York: Warner, 2005.

Calbom, Cherie, John Calbom, and Michael Mahaffey. *The Complete Cancer Cleanse*. Nashville, TN: Thomas Nelson, 2003.

Colbert, Don, M.D. *Toxic Relief: Restore Health and Energy Through Fasting and Detoxification*. Lake Mary, FL: Siloam, 2001 and 2003.

Lerner, Ben, D.C. "While you were sleeping." eNewsletter, issue 10, February 7, 2007. Maximizedliving@ecommunications.ca.

———. "Things you need to know about toxicity." eNewsletter, issue 14, March 6, 2007. Maximizedliving@ecommunications.ca.

Mercola, Joseph, M.D. http://www.mercola.com.

Morse, Robert, N.D. *The Detox Miracle Sourcebook*. Prescott, AZ: Holm Press, 2004.

Null, G., C. Dean, M. Feldman, D. Rasio, and D. Smith. "Death by Medicine," Life Extension Foundation, March 2004. http://www.lef.org/magazine/mag2004/mar2004_awsi_death_01.htm.

Saxon, V., N.D. "Chronic Fatigue Syndrome." Valerie Saxon's Silver Creek Labs.

Tortora, G., and S. Grabowski. *Introduction to the Human Body: The Essentials of Anatomy and Physiology*. Hoboken, NJ: John Wiley & Sons, 2004.

U.S. Environmental Protection Agency. "Endocrine Disruptor Screening Program." 1996. http://www.epa.gov/scipoly/oscpendo/pubs/edspoverview/background.htm.

Watson, Brenda. *Renew Your Life.* Clearwater, FL: Renew Life Press, 2002.

Whitney, M. T. "Prescription Drug Deaths Skyrocket 68 Percent Over Five Years As Americans Swallow More Pills." www.newstarget.com/021635.html, March 15, 2007. http://healthtruthrevealed.com/full-page.php?id=1119525302&&page=article.

CHAPTER FIVE

Calbom, Cherie, and John Calbom. *The Coconut Diet.* New York: Warner, 2005.

Calbom, Cherie, John Calbom, and Michael Mahaffey. *The Complete Cancer Cleanse.* Nashville, TN: Thomas Nelson, 2003.

Chao, A., M. J. Thun, C. J. Connell, M. L. McCullough, E. J. Jacobs, W. D. Flanders, C. Rodriguez, R. Sinha, and E. E. Calle. "Meat consumption and risk of colorectal cancer." *Journal of the American Medical Association* 293 (2005): 172–82. http://www.ncbi.nlm.nih.gov/entrez/query.fcgi?cmd=Retrieve&db=pubmed&dopt=Abstract&list_uids=15644544.

Colbert, Don, M.D. *Toxic Relief: Restore Health and Energy Through Fasting and Detoxification.* Lake Mary, FL: Siloam, 2001 and 2003.

Colon Cancer Alliance. "Disease Information: CRC Facts and Figures." http://www.ccalliance.org/about/disease/crcfacts.html.

Health-Science.com. "Intestinal Ecology." http://www.health-science.com/intestinal_health.html.

Jensen, B., D.C. *Tissue Cleansing Through Bowel Management.* Escondido, CA: Bernard Jensen Press, 1981.

MedicineWorld.org. "Colon Cancer Statistics." http://medicineworld.org/cancer/colon/stat.html.

Mercola, Joseph, M.D. http://www.mercola.com.

Morse, Robert, N.D. *The Detox Miracle Sourcebook.* Prescott, AZ: Holm Press, 2004.

Myers, D. "Colorectal Cancer Death Statistics for the U.S." http://coloncancer.about.com/od/cancerstatistics/a/US_Death_CRC.htm.

National Institute of Diabetes and Digestive and Kidney Diseases (NIDDK). "Constipation." http://www.digestive.niddk.nih.gov/ddiseases/pubs/constipation/index.htm.

———. "Diverticulosis and Diverticulitis." http://www.digestive.niddk.nih.gov/ddiseases/pubs/diverticulosis/.

Schultz, Richard. *Healing Colon Disease Naturally.* Marina del Rey, CA: Natural Healing Publications, 2003.

Watson, Brenda, N.D. *Essential Cleansing for Perfect Health.* Clearwater, FL: Renew Life Press, 2006.

———. *Renew Your Life.* Clearwater, FL: Renew Life Press, 2002.

Wikipedia. "Colorectal Cancer." http://en.wikipedia.org/wiki/Colorectal_cancer.

CHAPTER SIX

Anderson, Richard. *The Liver: Cleansing and Rejuvenating the Vital Organ.* Medford, OR: Christobe Publishing, 1999.

Calbom, Cherie, and John Calbom. *The Coconut Diet.* New York: Warner, 2005.

Calbom, Cherie, John Calbom, and Michael Mahaffey. *The Complete Cancer Cleanse.* Nashville, TN: Thomas Nelson, 2003.

National Institute of Diabetes and Digestive and Kidney Diseases (NIDDK). "Gallstones." http://digestive.niddk.nih.gov/ddiseases/pubs/gallstones/.

Schultz, Richard. *Healing Liver and Gallbladder Disease Naturally.* Marina del Rey, CA: Natural Healing Publications, 2003.

Watson, Brenda, N.D. *Essential Cleansing for Perfect Health.* Clearwater, FL: Renew Life Press, 2006.

CHAPTER SEVEN

Anderson, Richard. *Cleanse and Purify Thyself: Book* 1.5. Mt. Shasta, CA: Triumph Books, 1998.

Bergsson, Gudmundur, Jóhann Arnfinnsson, Ólafur Steingrímsson, and Halldor Thormar. "In Vitro Killing of Candida Albicans by Fatty Acids and Monoglycerides." *Antimicrobial Agents and Chemotherapy* 45, no. 11 (November 2001): 3209–3212. Institute of Biology, University of Iceland; Department of Anatomy, University of Iceland Medical School; and Department of Microbiology, National University Hospital in Reykjavik, Iceland.

Calbom, Cherie, and John Calbom. *The Coconut Diet.* New York: Warner, 2005.

Calbom, Cherie, John Calbom, and Michael Mahaffey. *The Complete Cancer Cleanse.* Nashville, TN: Thomas Nelson, 2003.

Cha, C. W. "A Study on the Effect of Garlic to Heavy Metal Poisoning of Rat." *Journal of Korean Medical Science* 2 (1987): 213–23. In *The Encyclopedia of Natural Medicine,* rev. 2nd ed., by Michael Murray and Joseph Pizzorno, Rocklin, CA: PrimaPublishing, 1998.

Clarkson, T. W., et al. "The prediction of intake of mercury vapor from amalgam," 247–264, in *Biological Monitoring of Toxic Metals,* New York: Plenum Press, 1988. Also *Dental Mercury Detox,* rev. ed., Sam Ziff, Michael Ziff, and Mats Hanson. Orlando, FL: Bio-Probe, Inc., 1988.

Colbert, Don, M.D. *Toxic Relief: Restore Health and Energy Through Fasting and Detoxification.* Lake Mary, FL: Siloam, 2001 and 2003.

Crook, William G., M.D. *The Yeast Connection.* Jackson, TN: Professional Books, 1983, 14.

DiagnoseMe.com. "Parasite Infection." http://www.diagnose-me.com/cond/C171466.html.

Gittleman, Ann Louise. *Natural Healing for Parasites.* New York: Healing Wisdom Publications, 1995.

Kroker, G. F. "Chronic Candidiasis and Allergy." In *Food Allergy and Intolerance,* edited by J. Brostoff and S. J. Challacombe. Philadelphia: W.B. Saunders, 1987, 850–72.

Mercola, Joseph, M.D. "Is Toxic Mercury Exposure Ruining Your Life?" http://www.mercola.com/2005/mar/9/mercury _exposure.htm.

Murray, Michael, N.D., and Joseph Pizzorno, N.D. *Encyclopedia of Natural Medicine.* Rocklin, CA: Prima Publishing, 1998, 306.

Naiman, Ingrid. "Parasitic Infection: Symptoms and Treatment,"KitchenDoctor.com.http://www.kitchendoctor.com/healthconditions/parasites/parasites.html.

Truss, O. *The Missing Diagnosis* (Birmingham, AL P.O. Box 26508, 1983) in Michael Murray, N.D. and Joseph Pizzorno, N.D. *Encyclopedia of Natural Medicine* (Rocklin, CA: Prima Publishing, 1998), 300.

Watson, Brenda, N.D. *Essential Cleansing for Perfect Health.* Clearwater, FL: Renew Life Press, 2006.

———. *Renew Your Life.* Clearwater, FL: Renew Life Press, 2002.

CHAPTER EIGHT

Bolt, Martin. *Pursuing Human Strengths.* New York: Worth Publishers, 2004.

Calbom, Cherie, John Calbom, and Michael Mahaffey. *The Complete Cancer Cleanse.* Nashville, TN: Thomas Nelson, 2003.

Cornell, Ann Weiser, Ph.D. *The Power of Focusing: A Practical Guide to Emotional Self-Healing.* New York: MJF Books, 1996.

Dwoskin, Dale, and Sedona Training Associates. *The Sedona Method Course Workbook: Your Keys to Lasting Happiness, Abundance and Well Being.* Sedona, AR: Sedona Training Associates, 1991–2000.

Holy Bible, New International Version. "Matthew 18:21–22." International Bible Society: Zondervan, 1984.

Hutchison, Michael. *Mega Brain Power: Transform Your Life with Mind Machines and Brain Nutrients.* New York: Hyperion, 1994.

Keyes, Ken, Jr. *Handbook to Higher Consciousness,* fifth ed. St. Mary, Kentucky: Cornucopia Institute, 1975.

Levine, Barbara Hobberman. *Your Body Believes Every Word You Say.* Boulder Creek, CA: Aslan Publishing, 1991.

Northrup, Christiane, M.D. *Women's Bodies, Women's Wisdom.* New York: Bantam, 1994.

Pert, Candace. *Molecules of Emotion.* New York: Simon & Schuster, 1999.

Sanford, Agnes. *The Healing Light.* New York: Ballantine Books, 1947.

Sanford, John, and Paula Sanford. *The Transformation of the Inner Man.* S. Plainfield, NJ: Bridge Publishing, Inc., 1982.

Soriano, Rino. "When Your Emotions Become Like Ticking Bombs and Cause Disease." http://www.ezinearticles.com.

Stokes, Hilary, M.S.W., M.A., and Kim Ward, M.A. "The Art of Forgiveness." *Sanoviv Health Retreat Healing Journal* 1991.

Tonsley, Cheryl, N.D. *Discovering Wholeness: The Spirit, Soul and Body Connection.* Littleton, CO: LFH Publishing, 2000.

Witvliet, Charlotte van Oyen, T. Ludwig, K. Vander Laan. "Granting Forgiveness or Harboring Grudges: Implications for Emotion, Physiology, and Health." *Psychological Science* 121 (2001): 117–23.

Wright, Henry. *A More Excellent Way.* Thomaston, GA: Pleasant Valley Publications, 1999.

Acknowledgments

To those who assisted in researching and writing this book, we are forever grateful.

Thank you to Michele Libin, who assisted us in researching and writing this book; we are so very appreciative. You are a dear friend and a valued writer with a wonderful future ahead; thank you for your great contribution to this project.

To our editors Diana Baroni and Leila Porteous, who made this project happen; thank you for your creativity and determination as always to make this book the very best it could be.

To our literary agent Pamela Harty, who once again helped us find a home for our work.

Lastly, we wish to express our deep and lasting appreciation to all the people, the Holy Trinity, and the angels who have assisted us with this book. To our dear heavenly Father, Jesus Christ, and Holy Spirit, thank You for guiding us throughout this project. We are so grateful that You showed us Your ways of wisdom and truth as to how to care for the human body. We feel that we've found the fountain of life in the juicing and cleansing programs we've been guided to embrace. Thank You for our health and the awesome responsibility of guiding those who have lost their health, peace of mind, or their way concerning the care of their bodies. For the healing You've given us and Your unconditional love, we are so very grateful.

Index

About the Authors

CHERIE CALBOM, M.S., is known as a leading expert on nutrition. She earned a master of science degree in nutrition from Bastyr University, where she now sits on the Board of Regents. She frequently appears on TV and speaks nationwide on the benefits of juicing and healthy living. She has written 16 previous books. Her best-selling book *Juicing for Life* has sold over 1.5 million copies. Cherie lives with her husband, John, in Edmonds, Washington.

JOHN CALBOM, M.A., is director of Trinity Retreat house, president of Trinity Wellness Institute, and a certified HeartMath provider. He is a behavioral medicine specialist, psychotherapist, and Eastern Orthodox priest. He was vice president of St. Luke Medical Center and worked as a behavioral medicine therapist in complementary and preventive medicine.